going Veggie

Published in the U.S. by
Ulysses Press
P.O. Box 3440
Berkeley, CA 94703
www.ulyssespress.com

ISBN: 978-1-61243-395-0
Library of Congress Control Number 2014943018

Printed in Korea by WE SP through Four Colour Print Group

10 9 8 7 6 5 4 3 2 1

Acquisitions Editor: Katherine Furman
Editor: Renee Rutledge
Proofreader: Lauren Harrison
Cover and Interior Design: Megan Wolf
Production: Jake Flaherty
Index: Sayre Van Young
Illustrations: pages 14, 73, 76, 82, 100, 106, 108, 118, 146, 170, 178 © Nikiparonak/ shutterstock.com; page 3 © bioraven/shutterstock.com; page 86 © rudall30/ shutterstock.com; page 124 © artspace/shutterstock.com

Distributed by Publishers Group West

IMPORTANT NOTE TO READERS: This book has been written and published strictly for informational and educational purposes only. It is not intended to serve as medical advice or to be any form of medical treatment. You should always consult your physician before altering or changing any aspect of your medical treatment and/ or undertaking a diet regimen, including the guidelines as described in this book. Do not stop or change any prescription medications without the guidance and advice of your physician. Any use of the information in this book is made on the reader's good judgment after consulting with his or her physician and is the reader's sole responsibility. This book is not intended to diagnose or treat any medical condition and is not a substitute for a physician.

This book is independently authored and published and no sponsorship or endorsement of this book by, and no affiliation with, any trademarked brands or other products mentioned within is claimed or suggested. All trademarks that appear in this book belong to their respective owners and are used here for informational purposes only. The author and publishers encourage readers to patronize the quality brands and products mentioned in this book.

going Veggie

THE 30-DAY GUIDE TO BECOMING A HEALTHY VEGETARIAN

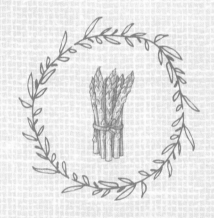

TRUDY SLABOSZ

THE CREATOR OF VEGGIENUMNUM.COM

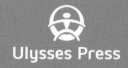

Ulysses Press

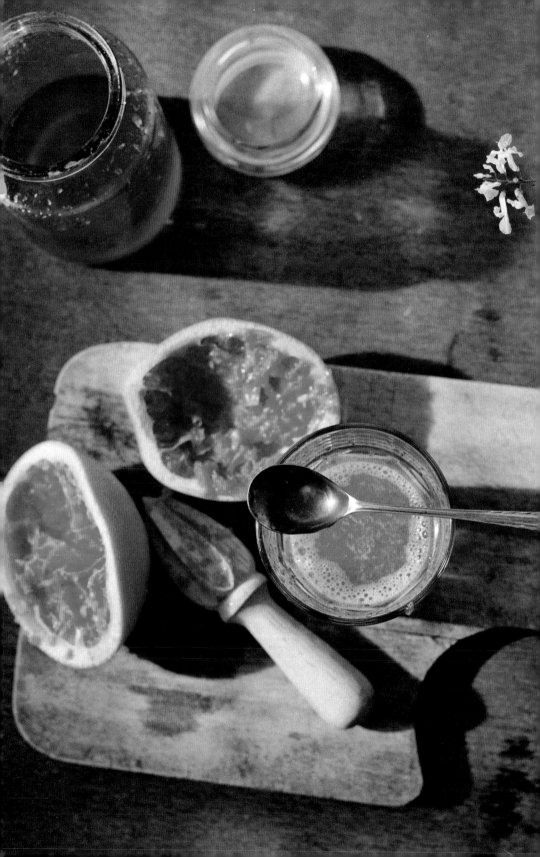

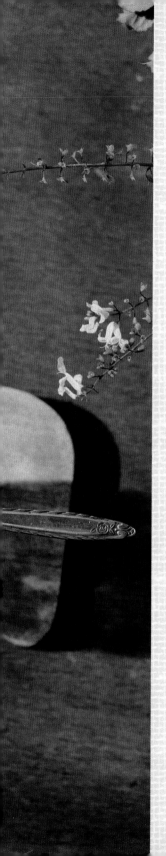

CONTENTS

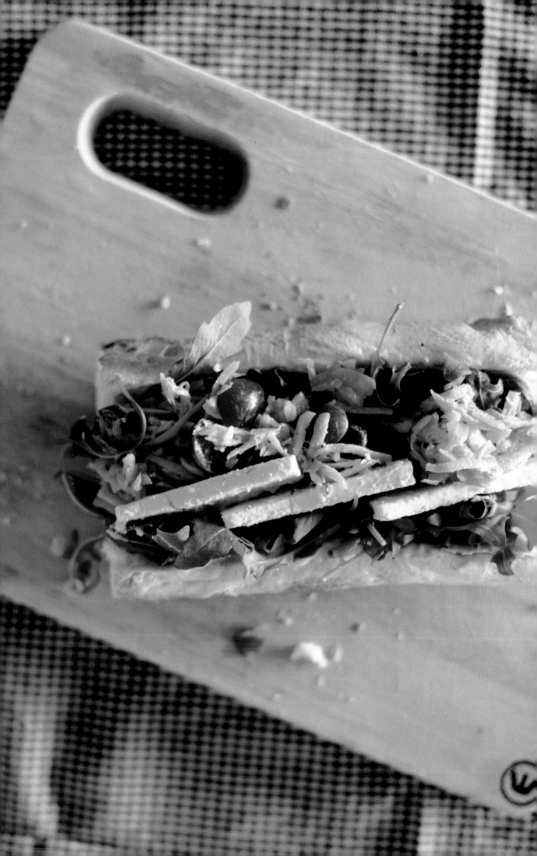

INTRODUCTION

Welcome to your healthy and happy journey into vegetarianism and the delicious world of vegetarian food. Within these pages you'll find everything you need to become the vegetarian you want to be—including easy-to-understand information on vegetarian nutrition, useful hints and tips on making the switch, and, most importantly, loads of recipes for nutritious, exciting, and delicious vegetarian food. Complete with a comprehensive 30-day meal guide, this book is for everyone, to be used every day, and it's all about helping you become a healthy and happy vegetarian.

A Note from the Author

For me, the decision to become a vegetarian was quite sudden. Even though I was raised as a meat-eater in a meat-eating family, I am lucky to have a wonderful mother—now a vegetarian herself—who regularly cooked us delicious veggie meals. Yet growing up, I never really considered becoming vegetarian. It was as a young adult that I came to the abrupt realization that I no longer wanted to eat meat, quite simply because I no longer wanted to eat animals. From that very day on, I've been on an amazing journey of constant discovery, driven by the enticing world of vegetarian food and the happiness I've found in my choice to be vegetarian.

It's a journey that's taken me from eating a terribly poor meat-free diet in those early days to one that now keeps me healthy and strong. It has inspired me to learn about nutrition and the different ingredients, flavors, and textures of food. It has truly sparked my love for the kitchen and a desire to be well nourished and well fed. Being vegetarian gets me cooking, creating wholesome meat-free meals to feed my young family, and inventing simple, tasty veggie foods to share with those I love. It brings me joy on many levels to live a compassionate life, and to discover how one simple choice can have such a waterfall effect has been remarkable.

I'm still learning every day, it's this journey of discovery and happiness that fueled my blog, *Veggie num num*. I wanted to create a place where everyone could find veggie inspiration, tips for whipping up wholesome good food, and lots of delicious recipes to cook and share with their family and friends. I believe that vegetarian food is for everyone, whether you choose to be completely vegetarian or not, and that everyone can cook and enjoy simple, healthy, and nourishing food—all it takes is a little inspiration.

An Introduction to Being Veggie

Choosing to be a vegetarian is all about the positives: the positive impact a plant-based diet can have on your health, on your approach to food and conscious eating, and on opening the door to an amazing bounty of delicious and wholesome ingredients. Far more than simply cutting meat from your diet, being a vegetarian can be a positive change for life, and the very best vegetarian you can be is a healthy and happy one.

Essentially, the single most important concept to grasp is that choosing to be vegetarian is much, much more than not eating meat. The very basis of vegetarian eating is a mindfulness of the food on your plate, and the best way to approach vegetarianism is to focus on what a vegetarian *does* eat, rather than what a vegetarian doesn't eat. It's this mindfulness that encourages healthy choices and a desire to seek out balanced, whole foods full of all the good stuff your body needs.

While the true definition of a vegetarian diet is one that doesn't include red meat, poultry, fish, shellfish, or animal-derived ingredients (find out more on page 42), in reality, each and every vegetarian is different. A vegetarian diet can range from strict vegetarian (i.e., vegan, which contains no meat, meat products, animal-derived ingredients, or animal products, including dairy, eggs, or honey) to a flexible-vegetarian diet, also known as flexitarianism, that includes some meat on occasion.

To be a truly healthy and happy vegetarian it's important to reach your own definition of what being veggie means and approach a meat-free diet at a pace and to an extent that's realistic to you. If becoming a strict vegetarian seems daunting, yet it's what you'd like to achieve, take a gradual approach by introducing a few meat-free meals a week and going from there. Or if you are just looking to change your diet for the better, don't impose strict limitations on yourself that may lead to failure. Instead consider cutting out only those animal products that are most important to your goals.

To what extent you embrace vegetarianism is entirely up to you and the secret to success is finding a healthy diet that fits in with your lifestyle and meets your individual dietary requirements. For more detailed advice on going veggie, plus loads of practical hints and tips on making the lifestyle change, turn to Chapter 2, "How to Become a Happy Veggie" on page 45.

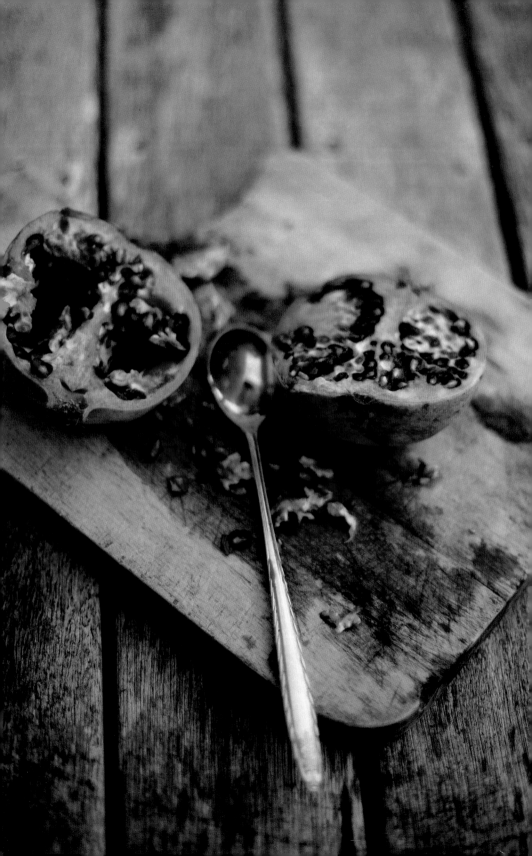

WHY CHOOSE TO BE VEGETARIAN?

It would be fair to say there are as many reasons people choose to be vegetarian as there are vegetarians. For some it's an acknowledgment of the conditions imposed on animals raised for food. Others adopt a meat-free diet for their health. Then there are those who make the choice because of religious, philosophical, or environmental motivation. It's important to embrace the reasons behind your own choice, as these are the very things that will keep you inspired and motivated along the way. Staying true to your own vegetarian values and personal definition of what that means will help you on your way to being a lifelong, happy veggie.

IS A VEGETARIAN DIET A HEALTHY CHOICE?

Following a well-balanced vegetarian diet is a healthy and positive choice for you and your body. Well-balanced, as in all healthy eating, comes down to moderation and variety: Eat foods in balanced proportions and enjoy a wide spectrum of nutritious foods each day. A meat-free diet can contain everything your body needs to stay fit, strong, healthy, and active. But even better than that, a healthy vegetarian diet includes far more of the good stuff—such as vegetables, fruits, grains, and legumes—providing a diet higher in beneficial fiber and antioxidants and with less of the saturated fat and cholesterol found in a typical Western diet.

It's important to be aware that there *can* be a higher risk of vitamin deficiencies, especially for vegans or those who do the potato-chips-and-pasta version of vegetarianism. By taking a little more care to eat the right foods in the right amounts, along with fortified foods and/or supplements for vegans, your diet can be a complete and satisfying one with little risk of vitamin deficiencies. The biggest health concern most new vegetarians have is adequate protein and iron intake, but rest assured there is a wide variety of delicious meat-free foods that offer a plant-based source of these and other essential vitamins and minerals. Vegans, who avoid dairy and eggs, need to take special care to include a reliable source of B12 (such as B12-fortified cereals, nondairy milks, faux-meat products, nutritional yeast, and/or a supplement), and all vegetarians should be sure to include lots of foods rich in protein, iron, zinc, and calcium. Have a look at the "Basic Vegetarian Nutrition" on page 20 to find out what foods are the very best sources of these essential nutrients. Plus read through "Maximize Your Food" on page 17 for lots of handy tips on including these nutrient-boosting foods in your everyday diet.

Whether you are a vegetarian or meat-eater, a healthy diet comes down to the individual and a willingness to eat the right foods for your body and overall well-being. Vegetarian or not, different life stages and lifestyles have different nutritional needs. If you are athletic, pregnant, lactating, or in adolescence, childhood, or old age, you can still thrive on a vegetarian diet; you just need to take special care to meet the additional dietary requirements of your body. The most important thing to remember when considering a change in diet is that everybody has differing nutritional needs, and if you have any concerns about meeting healthy requirements for your own body, you should seek professional advice.

For more detailed information on vegetarian nutrition and which foods to include in your vegetarian diet, have a read through "The Healthy Veggie" chapter on page 15.

SO, WHAT DOES A VEGETARIAN EAT? IS IT ALL SOGGY LENTILS AND BORING TOFU?

As a new vegetarian you may worry about what you're going to eat now that your diet is meat-free, and in a society where most traditional meals are based around meat, this is understandable. Fundamental to being a happy veggie is realizing that a vegetarian meal is not simply what you used to cook with the meat taken out.

Meat and meat products are only a small portion of the ever-growing variety of foods available today. With an abundance and variety of fresh vegetables, fruits, grains, cereals, nuts, seeds, and faux-meat vegetarian options at your fingertips, preparing interesting and delicious meat-free meals couldn't be easier or more fun!

There's no better way to start enjoying an appetizing veggie diet than to get cooking. Enjoying exciting vegetarian food is all about combining different textures and flavors and using healthy, whole food ingredients to create tasty meals that just happen to be meat-free. This book offers loads of information on the variety of vegetarian foods, how to include them in your diet, and, of course, all the veggie recipes for delicious mealtime inspiration.

Be a Healthy, Happy Veggie

Ultimately, being a healthy and happy vegetarian means discovering a huge variety of delicious and wholesome ingredients, embracing a wholly positive approach to food and diet, and appreciating the resulting effect this has on conscious eating, health, and well-being. It's about making a positive choice for your own body, the planet, and the lives of animals. And the very best news is that vegetarian food is normal food—it's satisfying, nutritious, and just as easy to prepare. With a little sense of adventure and lots of tasty inspiration, you'll soon discover the joys of being veggie.

For those unsure of where to start, simply set the goal of becoming your own vegetarian, guided by your own choices and the needs of your own body and lifestyle. There's no rush to cut all the meat and animal products from your diet; take things at a pace and to an extent that fits within the pattern of your life and ideals. Don't beat yourself up if you want a steak—it takes time to discover the abundant world of vegetarian food, and it's more important to enjoy the journey than deprive yourself along the way.

Being vegetarian is being a conscious eater—acknowledging where the food on your plate has come from and making the conscious choice to eat those foods that nourish your body. Healthy food choices can have a remarkably positive impact on your overall well-being, regardless of if you are vegetarian or not. Enjoy the happiness and good health that comes from filling your belly with good food and your body with wholesome nutrition. Cook with love, for those you love, and with those foods you love to eat. That's what makes a happy and healthy vegetarian!

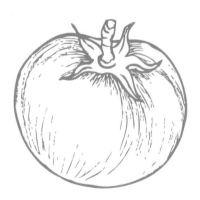

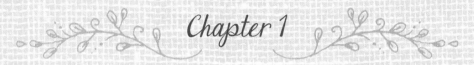

Chapter 1

THE HEALTHY VEGGIE

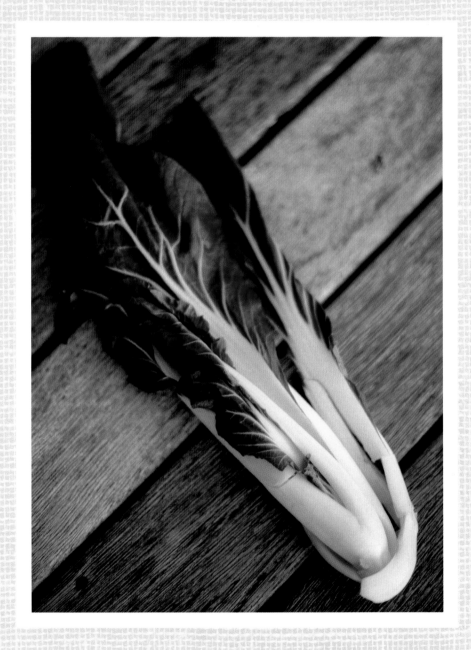

Whether you eat meat or are vegetarian, learning what foods are the very best for your body can make all the difference in ensuring good health and a long, happy life.

Your diet influences your overall health and well-being in countless ways. Eating the right foods will promote strong immunity and a healthy digestive system, boost your cognitive abilities, and provide lots of energy to keep you feeling fit, strong, and active. A poor diet can contribute to a host of ailments—from lethargy, digestive disorders, vitamin deficiencies, and weak immunity to more serious illnesses like heart disease and type 2 diabetes. As the old saying goes, you are what you eat. For a healthy vegetarian this is just as, if not more, relevant.

The simplest way to approach good nutrition is to understand that your body needs a variety of nutrients to function properly, and the foods you eat contain them in varying degrees. Choosing the very best food for your body can be easy. All it takes is a little knowledge of the very best sources of vegetarian foods containing essential vitamins and minerals to include in your everyday diet. In this chapter you'll find everything you need to navigate the world of nutrient-rich, plant-based food. Plus, discover the role different nutrients play in overall health and, most importantly, how to adopt these foods into your everyday diet.

Variety for Vitality

Plant-based foods offer a diverse and rich supply of essential nutrients—the key is to eat a balanced diet packed with a variety of delicious fresh fruits, vegetables, whole-grains, legumes, soy products, nuts, and seeds. Aim to include a varied combination of these foods each day to maximize your essential nutrient intake.

Eating a range of different types of foods can be easy. Start by adding various seeds, nuts, and dried fruits to your breakfast cereal. Mix and match a variety of leafy greens in your salads, such as baby kale, spinach, beet greens, and arugula. Give your dinner a nutritional boost by adding quinoa to rice and barley to soups. See every meal as an opportunity to add flavor, texture, and goodness to your diet through healthy, fresh, and whole-food ingredients.

A Rainbow on Your Plate

The vibrant colors of fruit, vegetables, herbs, and spices signify the rich and diverse range of beneficial antioxidants, vitamins, and minerals they contain. A simple and tasty way to ensure you're packing lots of different nutrients into your diet is to have lots of color on your plate. Choose bright reds, oranges, greens, purples, and yellows—a colorful plate not only tastes great, it's also the very best for you.

Raw salads and vegetable dishes offer a simple way to introduce lots of colors to your diet. Plus, fresh fruit smoothies and vegetable juices are a tasty and nutritious solution to pumping up your daily intake of colorful foods. Check out "Smoothies & Juices" on page 73 for some inspiration.

Maximize Your Food

There are a number of things you can do when sourcing, storing, and cooking your food that will ensure you enjoy their full nutritional value.

Always choose the freshest produce. In-season fruit and vegetables are the best. Consider visiting your local farmer's market for the freshest local and seasonal produce. If you can't get fresh, use frozen rather than canned—frozen fruit and vegetables usually have nearly the same nutritional value as their fresh counterparts.

Buying fruit and vegetables in season means you're getting the freshest, tastiest, and cheapest produce all year round. The chart on page 19 is a brief guide to eating through the seasons. As the season changes, let your diet follow—it's a great way to enjoy a large variety of different foods and flavors throughout the year.

Store fresh foods correctly. Keep ripe fruits and all your leafy greens, sprouts, softer vegetables, and anything that's been cut or cold stored in your crisper drawer and use within a few days. Leave fruits to ripen in the pantry along with tomatoes and avocados. Most unripe fruit will not ripen properly if stored in the fridge.

Leave skins on. Most of your fresh food's nutritional value is in or just under the skin. Wash and/or scrub your fruit and vegetables instead of peeling them, whenever possible.

Steam, grill, or roast your vegetables instead of boiling or microwaving. Boiling and microwaving vegetables can damage their nutritional content and flavor. Steaming, grilling, and roasting them brings out their best flavors while maintaining most of their nutrients.

Eat your veggies raw. Raw vegetables are the very best when it comes to nutritional value. Try to include lots of raw veggies in your diet with fresh juices, snacks, and salads.

Save your good oils. Keep the good oils like olive, flax, walnut, and pumpkin seed for dressings and sauces, and use rice bran, peanut, and sunflower oils for cooking.

FRUITS & VEGETABLES BY SEASON

Summer

Apricots	Cucumbers	Melons	Strawberries
Beets/Beet greens	Eggplant	Nectarines	Tomatoes
Bell peppers	Figs	Peaches	Zucchini
Blueberries	Grapes	Peas	
Carrots	Lemons	Plums	
Corn	Limes	Radishes	

Fall/Autumn

Apples	Celery	Pears	Raspberries
Beets	Eggplant	Persimmons	Spinach
Broccoli	Fennel	Plums	Sweet potatoes
Brussels sprouts	Garlic	Pomegranate	Swiss chard
Cabbage	Ginger	Potatoes	Turnips
Carrots	Leeks	Pumpkin	
Cauliflower	Mushrooms	Radicchio	

Winter

Broccoli	Celery root/Celeriac	Kiwifruit	Potatoes
Brussels sprouts	Collards	Leeks	Pumpkin
Butternut squash	Fennel	Oranges	Sweet potatoes
Clementines/Mandarins	Grapefruit	Parsnips	Tamarillos
Cabbages	Kale	Pomegranates	Turnips
Cauliflower			

Spring

Apricots	Celery root/Celeriac	Green beans	Oranges
Artichokes	Cucumber	Kale	Peas
Asparagus	Fava beans/Broad beans	Leeks	Spinach
Broccoli	Grapefruit	Lemons	Strawberries
		Limes	Watercress

Limit processed foods. Full of the things you don't need (additives and preservatives) and lacking in the things you do, processed foods offer little nutritional value and are often higher in refined sugar, fats, and salt.

Choose predominately whole-grains. Look for whole-grain choices when it comes to breads, pasta, cereals, and rice. Whole-grains are just that, whole, and are a far superior source of fiber, vitamins, and minerals.

Basic Vegetarian Nutrition

All foods contain a varying degree and combination of nutrients. Our bodies need these nutrients to function, repair cells, and maintain overall health. A diverse and wholesome meat-free diet should contain a wealth of essential vitamins and minerals, typically with far less saturated fat and cholesterol and much more of the good stuff like fiber, folic acid, and antioxidants.

Note: Nutritional information provided here is a general guide only and not a complete guide to essential vitamins and minerals or a substitute for professional nutritional or medical advice. When switching to a plant-based diet, it can be a great idea to seek the advice of a nutritionist or doctor, especially if you have specific nutritional requirements, medical needs, questions, or concerns.

As a quick reference guide, the following section details key essential nutrients followed by a list of the best vegetarian sources in which to find them. For more information on the different types of vegetarian foods listed here and tips on how to include these in your vegetarian diet, read through "Maximize Your Food" on page 17 or check out the glossary on page 187.

PROTEIN

Protein is vital for growth, cell repair, and maintaining optimal health. Some new vegetarians may wonder about vegetarian sources of protein; animal products like dairy and eggs offer a ready source of complete protein (containing all nine essential amino acids; see below). Vegans and all vegetarians should look to a variety of plant-based foods to enjoy a complete high-quality protein diet. There are lots of delicious and nutritious vegetarian protein sources, and it's by eating a good variety and combination of the following foods throughout your day that you'll meet your body's complete protein needs.

Amino acids are the building blocks of protein. While your body is able to manufacture most of the amino acids it needs to maintain optimal health, nine must be acquired from the foods you eat, making them essential to your diet. (These are histidine, isoleucine, leucine, methionine, phenylalanine, threonine, tryptophan, valine, and lysine.) Not all protein-rich foods are complete protein foods containing all nine essential amino acids. Yet eating a varied combination of plant-based protein foods each day provides a variety of these nine essential amino acids that your body can combine. For vegetarians, a diet rich in an assortment of protein-rich, plant-based foods such as legumes, soy, whole grains, nuts, and seeds will easily provide your body with a source of complete protein. Be sure to eat a variety of the following foods throughout the day—combinations like beans or soybeans with rice or seeds and nuts with whole-grains are ideal for obtaining all nine essential amino acids in your diet.

- Dairy products
- Edamame
- Free-range eggs
- Legumes (beans and lentils)
- Nutritional yeast
- Nuts, primarily almonds, pistachios, pine nuts, and pecans

- Seeds, primarily chia, hemp, pumpkin, sunflower, and sesame
- Soy products (tofu and tempeh)
- Spirulina
- Whole-grains, primarily amaranth, barley, buckwheat, oats, and quinoa

CALCIUM

Vital for the healthy growth and maintenance of bones and for brain function, calcium is fundamental to a healthy diet. Although dairy products are the popular source of calcium, the following assorted plant-based and fortified foods provide a ready source of it for vegetarians and vegans.

- Blackstrap molasses
- Calcium-fortified breakfast cereals
- Calcium-fortified, dairy-free milks like soy, rice, oat, and almond
- Calcium-fortified tofu (simply check the ingredients)
- Dairy products
- Dried fruits, primarily figs and apricots
- Green, leafy vegetables, primarily broccoli and kale
- Nuts, primarily Brazil nuts, almonds, and nut butters made from these
- Seeds, primarily sesame seeds and tahini

IRON

Iron assists the lungs in carrying oxygen throughout the body and promotes resistance to disease and infection. Aside from protein, adequate iron intake is probably what many new vegetarians worry about the most. There are, however, many plant-based sources of iron, and by eating a well-balanced diet that includes a variety of the following foods and plenty of vitamin C (best consumed with the iron-rich foods), your iron intake can match those of a typical, non-vegetarian diet.

- Blackstrap molasses
- Dried fruits, primarily apricots, prunes, and peaches
- Edamame
- Green, leafy vegetables
- Iron-fortified foods like breakfast cereals
- Legumes (beans and lentils)
- Nuts, primarily almonds, pine nuts, pistachios, and hazelnuts
- Raw cacao (available as nibs and powder)
- Seeds, primarily pumpkin seeds, sesame seeds, and tahini
- Spirulina
- Whole-grains, primarily amaranth, oats, quinoa, and spelt

ZINC

Zinc supports the body's ability to heal and promotes a healthy immune system.

- Legumes (beans and lentils)
- Nuts, primarily cashews and almonds
- Seeds, primarily sunflower and sesame
- Tofu and fermented soy products (tempeh, miso)
- Wheat germ
- Zinc-fortified breakfast cereals

VITAMIN A

Vitamin A promotes resistance to infection and supports healthy skin, bones, teeth, and eyes.

- Dairy products
- Green, leafy vegetables, primarily broccoli, spinach, and arugula
- Yellow/orange fruits and vegetables, fresh or dried (sweet potatoes, carrots, apricots, cantaloupe, mangos, and peaches)

B GROUP VITAMINS

The B group vitamins—thiamin, riboflavin, niacin, pantothenic acid, folate, and vitamin B6—play an important role in energy metabolism and nerve function.

- Bananas
- Green, leafy vegetables
- Legumes, primarily lentils, chickpeas, navy beans, and kidney beans
- Mushrooms
- Nutritional yeast
- Nuts, primarily almonds, chestnuts, hazelnuts, peanuts, pecans, and pistachios
- Seeds, primarily pumpkin, sesame, and sunflower
- Sweet potato
- Whole-grains, primarily barley, brown rice, and oats

VITAMIN C

Promoting resistance to infection and stimulating the immune system, vitamin C also works to support healthy bones, skin, and red blood cells. Importantly, vitamin C assists the body in efficient iron absorption, so throw in some vitamin C–rich foods when consuming an iron-rich meal.

- Fruits, primarily citrus, berries, kiwifruit, tomatoes, and avocado
- Vegetables, primarily potato, cauliflower, and red bell pepper

IODINE

Important for hormonal development, iodine is essential to metabolic function and a healthy thyroid gland.

- Dairy
- Fennel
- Free-range eggs
- Potato (with skins)
- Spinach
- Seaweed

CARBOHYDRATES

Carbohydrates provide fuel for the body to function and energy for physical and mental activity. Complex carbohydrates from whole-grains are preferable over simple carbohydrates from refined grains, like white rice and white bread, as they offer greater nutritional value with added fiber, vitamins, and minerals. Fruits and vegetables also provide abundant levels of carbohydrates and are a good source of energy for the body.

- Fruits, primarily bananas
- Legumes (beans and lentils)
- Vegetables, primarily potatoes, sweet potatoes, pumpkin, zucchini, peas, and corn
- Whole-grains

FIBER

Fiber plays an essential role in maintaining a healthy digestive system.

- Dried fruits, primarily apple, apricot, pears, and raisins
- Fruits, primarily berries, oranges, kiwifruit, and pears
- Legumes (beans and lentils)
- Tempeh
- Vegetables, primarily green and leafy vegetables, cabbage, carrots, and cauliflower
- Whole-grains, primarily barley and wheat

FATS

Good fats are fundamental to maintaining optimal health and especially important in the support of brain and nerve function, aiding mental concentration and memory while keeping your skin hydrated and healthy.

- Avocados
- Olives and olive oil
- Nuts, primarily almonds, peanuts, macadamias, pecans, and walnuts, as well as butters and oils made from them
- Seeds, primarily flaxseed, pumpkin, sunflower, and sesame, as well as butters and oils made from them

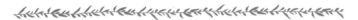

IMPORTANT NUTRIENTS FOR VEGETARIANS

OMEGA-3 FATTY ACIDS. Omega-3 is an important nutrient essential for healthy brain and heart function. As fish is often the common source for non-vegetarians, it can be lacking in a vegetarian diet without inclusion of the following foods.

- Chia seeds
- Flaxseeds (linseeds), also available as flax oil and flax meal
- Hemp seeds and hemp seed oil

VITAMIN B12. Vitamin B12 is an essential nutrient vital to healthy brain and nerve function. Strict vegetarians who avoid dairy and eggs must be sure to eat B12-fortified foods or include a B12 supplement to meet dietary requirements.

- B12-fortified cereals
- B12-fortified nondairy milks
- B12 supplement
- Dairy products
- Free-range eggs
- Nutritional yeast (check that the one you buy is fortified with B12)
- Sesame seeds and tahini
- Walnuts and walnut butter and oil

VITAMIN D. When exposed to adequate daily sunlight, the body makes vitamin D, important for bone health and defense against disease. If you are restricted by lifestyle or live in a climate where sun exposure is at a minimum, be sure to include the following foods in your diet.

- Free-range eggs
- Vitamin D–fortified milks and cereals

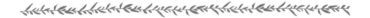

The Veggie Pantry

Discovering the wonderfully diverse world of vegetarian food is the foundation of a truly healthy and happy veggie. A balanced meat-free diet can contain everything your body needs to be healthy, strong, and active—the key is to eat a varied combination of the right foods each day for your optimal health and well-being.

There are five main groups of foods that make up a complete vegetarian diet: whole grains; vegetables; legumes and soy products; fruits; and nuts and seeds. In addition to these, some vegetarians may also include dairy and/or eggs. A balanced combination of these foods in your diet should allow you to meet your dietary requirements, plus enjoy a wealth of delicious and nutritious ingredients.

A well-stocked pantry is the key to preparing interesting and nutritious foods. Plus, you'll have lots of ingredients at the ready for simple, quick, and delicious meals when time is short. Fortunately, shopping for your vegetarian diet is much like shopping for any healthy diet, with plenty of fresh fruits and vegetables, rice, pasta, grains, nuts, seeds, sauces, spices, and other goodies on the list. Try to keep a good supply of healthy foods and basic elements for delicious dishes on hand and shop in a variety of places to ensure you get fresh and authentic ingredients.

The following information is a guide to key vegetarian foods, vegetarian pantry staples, and a well-balanced vegetarian diet. It provides lots of basic nutritional information, suggested servings per day, plus a guide to the best sources and tips on how to easily include these foods in your diet. This is a good list of basic standby ingredients—veggie pantry items you'll use every day in a variety of dishes. (You can find a detailed glossary on more unusual ingredients on page 187.)

The servings per day listed in this chapter are a general guide only and are by no means strict medical advice. Your ideal daily nutrient and calorie intake will vary according to your gender, daily physical activity, and age. Be sure to adapt these guidelines to meet your personal nutritional needs and lifestyle and, as always, seek professional medical or nutritional advice if you have any concerns or specific health requirements (particularly those pregnant or lactating, or in childhood, adolescence, or advanced age).

GRAINS AND CEREALS

Nutrient-dense and filling, grains and cereals are a key element to any healthy vegetarian diet.

They're high in fiber, B vitamins, and complex carbohydrates. They offer a good source of zinc, iron, and protein while providing your body with an important, nutrient-rich supply of energy. A large variety of whole grains and whole-grain products are now available from your natural foods store and, more recently, the supermarket. Eating whole-grain products doesn't mean you have to cut white rice and pasta out of your diet completely—simply add in more whole-grain choices and mix it up a little with the wealth of healthy ingredients now readily available.

Aim for around 5+ servings/day. One serving equals one of the following:

- ½ cup cooked of pasta, rice, or whole-grain (barley, buckwheat, quinoa, etc.)
- 1 slice of whole wheat bread
- 1 cup of cereal
- 1 small whole wheat muffin
- 3–4 whole-grain crackers

The following grains are good nutrient-dense sources:

- Barley
- Black rice
- Brown rice (puffed rice and brown rice crackers)
- Buckwheat (raw or toasted groats, puffed buckwheat and buckwheat flour and pasta)
- Bulgur
- Cornmeal (polenta)
- Millet
- Noodles (soba, udon, and rice)
- Oats (rolled oats, steel-cut oats, and oat flour)
- Quinoa (and quinoa pasta, flakes, flour, crackers, and bread)
- Rye (rolled rye, rye flour, and rye bread)
- Spelt (and rolled spelt, spelt flour, and spelt pasta)
- White rice (basmati, arborio, and short grain)
- Whole wheat and multigrain flours and products made from these (crackers, bread, buns, muffins, tortillas, and pita bread)
- Whole wheat couscous
- Whole wheat pasta
- Wild rice

TIPS Switch out refined-grain products like white bread and wheat pasta for multigrain breads and whole wheat, spelt, or buckwheat pasta. Try adding cooked and cooled barley, buckwheat, or quinoa to your salads, and puffed buckwheat, rolled spelt, or quinoa flakes to your breakfast cereal; eat whole-grain crackers, rice cakes, and cereals throughout the day. Plus, check out all the recipes in this book for lots of delicious inspiration on cooking with whole grains and whole-grain products.

Whole Grains

Keep a good selection of different whole-grains on hand to mix up your diet and add texture and flavor to your meals. Look for raw buckwheat, quinoa, millet, and barley, which can be cooked according to the packet instructions and served either hot or cold, much the same as rice and pasta. Couscous and bulgur are ideal quick-fix ingredients to use in salads or vegetable dishes. Keep some coarse cornmeal on hand for preparing delicious polenta. Try shopping in natural foods stores and buy a variety of whole grains in bulk. Most will store for long periods in a well-sealed jar or container in your pantry.

Cereals

There's a host of cereals readily available from your supermarket or natural foods store. Try puffed buckwheat; amaranth and rice; quinoa and whole wheat flakes; and rye and spelt oats—great for adding to homemade granola, porridge mixes, cookies, cakes, and muffins. Nearly all cereals will keep for long periods when stored in a well-sealed jar or container.

Rice

Rice is an essential component to many wholesome meals and stores well for long periods in a sealed container. Depending on the dish, there are a few common types of rice that are good to have on hand. Brown rice is both nutritious and versatile, with a lovely nutty flavor—it teams well with curries and roasted vegetables and is beautiful in salad dishes. Wild rice and black rice are nutritious and make for unusual additions to soups, salads, and warm rice bowls. Try black rice in soups and puddings, and use wild rice for salads. Basmati is lovely with curry and other spicy dishes, and because the grains don't stick together, it's perfect for pilafs. Look for arborio rice to use in risotto and jasmine for Asian-style dishes. The versatility and muted flavor of short grain rice make it a favorite for sushi, rice puddings, and desserts.

Pasta

There is now a vast selection of different pastas, from wheat to spelt and buckwheat, available at your natural foods store or on the supermarket shelves. There are also gluten-free varieties, often with a combination of different grains, including rice, quinoa, and corn. Speedy to prepare, pasta makes a great standby to have in your pantry. Keep a selection stored in sealed containers for quick meal solutions. Choose thick pasta like fettuccine for robust or creamy sauces, thin spaghettis for oil-based sauces, and shapes like penne and spiral pasta for chunky sauces and baked pasta dishes.

Noodles

Noodles make an excellent addition to soups, stir-fries, and salads. Many are super quick to prepare, taking only a few minutes to boil, which means they are perfect for a quick and nutritious meal. Look for thick or thin rice noodles for use in stir-fries and soba, udon, and ramen noodles for soups, salads, and other quick meals. Let's not forget bean thread noodles, also called cellophane or vermicelli noodles, perfect for salads and rice paper rolls.

Flours

With a good variety of different flours now available at your natural foods store and supermarket, it's a great idea to keep a selection on hand. Try a mix of buckwheat and plain flour in pancakes, or add spelt or amaranth to cookie or muffin recipes. Be sure to have plain and self-rising flours on hand for all your baking and batter needs, and try mixing it up with buckwheat, rye, spelt, chickpea, amaranth, quinoa, and more. Many whole-grain flours will have a shorter shelf life than refined flour does. Keep them stored in a sealed container in your pantry or, alternatively, in your freezer.

VEGETABLES

By far one of the healthiest foods you can eat, vegetables offer a powerful and diverse range of vitamins and minerals, including B vitamins, vitamins A and C, iron, calcium, and fiber. To get the very best from your veggies, choose the freshest produce; eat them raw, steamed, grilled, or baked; keep their skins on (where possible); and aim for a good variety each day. Packaged frozen vegetables offer a good backup to fresh veggies and are a convenient standby to have in your freezer for a quick meal.

Aim for around 5+ servings/day. One serving equals one of the following:

- 1 cup diced raw vegetables
- ½ cup cooked vegetables
- ¾ cup fresh juiced vegetables

The following vegetables are good nutrient-dense sources:

- Beets and beet greens
- Broccoli
- Cabbage
- Carrots
- Cauliflower
- Celery
- Cucumbers
- Eggplant
- Fennel
- Garlic
- Ginger
- Green beans
- Kale
- Leeks
- Mushrooms
- Onions
- Peas
- Peppers
- Potatoes
- Spinach and other green leafy vegetables
- Squash (like pumpkin)
- Sweet potatoes
- Tomatoes

Along with grains and cereals, vegetables should form the basis of your vegetarian diet. Be sure to eat plenty of salads, vegetable dishes, stir-fries, and curries loaded with a variety of vegetables. Fresh juices are another great way to add extra veggie power to you daily diet; or, try vegetable sticks for snacking—raw carrot, cucumber, and peppers are great with some hummus for dipping. Check out the "Snacks" and "Smoothies & Juices" sections, as well as all the recipes, to find lots of inspiration for pumping up your vegetable intake.

LEGUMES AND SOY

Canned or dried legumes (beans and lentils) are an excellent pantry standby, and there's a vast variety readily available to purchase in supermarkets and often in bulk from natural foods stores. Canned beans offer a handy and quick option as they require no presoak or cooking—simply drain and rinse well before use. Preparation times vary for dried beans, but most should be presoaked for 8–12 hours, and then cooked for up to 60 minutes, depending on the variety. Most lentils do not need presoaking and their cooking time is remarkably less, usually 25–45 minutes. Prepared beans and lentils are great thrown into anything from curries and roasted vegetable dishes to soups and salads.

An invaluable and versatile source of vegetarian protein, many legumes also offer a source of calcium and iron, making them an incredibly useful and nutritious addition to your vegetarian diet. Providing a good supply of high-quality carbohydrates, fiber, zinc, and B vitamins, along with other essential nutrients, legumes are a staple in many vegetarian dishes.

Legumes are ideal as a simple substitute to meat in your favorite dishes. A good starting point is to experiment with the huge variety of bean or lentil burgers, sausages, and faux-meats readily available from your natural foods store or supermarket. Look for those that are minimally processed and contain zero or few additives and preservatives. And, check out the recipes or the information on what to eat when you feel like something familiar (page 50) for lots of inspiration and ideas on including nutritious legumes in your diet.

Soy products offer a great source of lean protein—being both low in saturated fat and cholesterol they make an excellent substitute to meat in many vegetarian meals. Importantly, especially for vegans, choose calcium-fortified tofu (check the ingredients label) and look for soy milk fortified with calcium (some will also have added B12 or vitamin D).

Soy foods, such as tofu and tempeh, are incredibly versatile and make up a majority of the meat alternatives readily available in your supermarket. Look for firm tofu to use in stir-fries and curries, and silken tofu for sauces, desserts, dressings, and soups. Try marinated tofu for use in salads and quick meals. Tempeh is great as a replacement for chicken and beef in anything from soups to stir-fries and burgers. For an easy vegetarian meal that seems familiar, test out the huge variety of vegetarian soy-based burgers, sausages, and ground meat—great on their own or as a substitute to meat in cooking. Soy milk, as well as soy-based cheese and yogurt also offer a handy plant-based alternative to their dairy counterparts.

Aim for around 3 servings/day. One serving equals one of the following:

- ½ cup cooked beans, peas, or lentils

- ½ cup tofu, tempeh, or product made from these (tofu sausage, burger, etc.)
- 1 cup soy milk or yogurt

The following legumes and soy products are good nutrient-dense sources:

- Beans (cannellini beans, butter beans, kidney beans, navy and pinto beans, etc.)
- Chickpeas
- Edamame
- Faux-meats (vegetarian burgers, sausages, ground meat, etc.) made from tofu or tempeh

- Faux-meats (vegetarian burgers, sausages, ground meat, etc.) made from beans or lentils
- Lentils (red, brown, and puy)
- Miso paste (fermented soy)
- Soy milk and soy yogurt
- Split peas
- Tempeh
- Tofu

TIPS

Experiment with the variety of soy burgers, sausages, and faux-meats readily available from your natural foods store or supermarket. Look for those that are minimally processed and contain zero or few additives and preservatives. And check out the recipes or the information on what to eat when you feel like something familiar (page 50) for lots of inspiration and ideas on including nutritious soy products in your diet.

FRUIT

A super source of antioxidants and fiber, fresh fruit hydrates and provides energy, along with a host of vitamins and minerals, for the body. Again, choose the freshest seasonal produce and leave the skins on things like apples, pears, kiwifruit, and plums for optimal nutrient value. Dried fruits offer a good source of fiber and are a convenient item stored in your pantry to throw in salads, breakfast cereals, or your lunch box.

Aim for around 3 servings/day. One serving equals one of the following:

- 1 whole medium-sized fruit (apple, banana, pear, or orange)
- ¾ cup fresh-squeezed fruit juice (neither pre-bottled nor from concentrate)
- 1 cup diced fresh fruit or berries
- ¼ cup dried fruit (look for those that are preservative-free and with no added sugar)

The following fruits are good nutrient-dense sources:

- Apples
- Apricots (and dried apricots)
- Avocados
- Bananas
- Berries (blueberries, blackberries, raspberries, strawberries)
- Dates
- Figs (and dried figs)
- Grapefruit
- Kiwifruit
- Mangos
- Melons
- Oranges
- Papaya
- Pears
- Plums

TIPS Fruit makes the perfect snack—it's portable, fresh, healthy, and full of fiber and energy for your body. Pack an apple, banana, or cup of berries or chopped fruit for your midmorning snack. Smoothies and fresh juices are another great way to enjoy lots of different fruits. Avoid packaged juices, as these are often high in sugar with little to no nutritional content—instead check out "Smoothies & Juices" on page 73 for inspiration on making your own.

NUTS AND SEEDS

Nuts and seeds are some of the most nutrient-dense foods and are a great source of vegetarian protein, iron, zinc, and many other essential vitamins and minerals. Walnuts, flaxseeds, sesame seeds, and chia seeds also offer an important source of omega-3 fatty acids. As most seeds and nuts are a rich source of fats, although predominantly good-for-you fats, it's best to limit them to 1–2 servings a day.

Whole nuts and seeds keep well stored in jars or containers and are great for a quick snack or adding a nutritional boost to nearly every meal. Raw or dry roasted nuts are the best—avoid salted and sweetened varieties. There are many great seed mixes available from your natural foods store or in the health aisle of the supermarket. And be sure to keep ground nuts and seeds in the fridge, as they can go rancid otherwise. Look for chia, sunflower, sesame, and pumpkin seeds, and stock up on raw almonds, pistachios, Brazil nuts, and more. Nut and seed butters are super handy to have in the pantry—always choose those that contain no added sugar, salt, or other additives, or even better, make your own. A good combination to look out for is ABC (almond, Brazil nut, and cashew butter). Plus, have some tahini (sesame seed paste) on hand for whipping up dressings, sauces, and hummus, using in smoothies, or spreading on toast, sandwiches, and wraps.

TIPS Nuts and seeds are easy to add to your everyday diet. Throw a serving of seeds or chopped nuts or a drizzle of tahini in your salad or morning bowl of oatmeal. There are many nut butters now available on the shelves at your natural foods store or supermarket—try some spread on whole-grain toast for breakfast or add a spoonful to your daily smoothie.

Aim for around 1–2 servings/day. One serving equals one of the following:

- ¼ cup nuts
- ¼ cup seeds
- 1–2 tablespoons nut and/or seed butter

The following nuts and seeds are good nutrient-dense sources:

- Almonds
- Brazil nuts
- Cashews
- Chia seeds
- Flaxseeds, also available as flax meal or flax oil
- Hazelnuts
- Hemp seeds
- Pecans
- Pine nuts
- Pistachios
- Pumpkin seeds
- Sesame seeds and tahini
- Sunflowers seeds
- Walnuts

DAIRY

Although not part of a vegan diet, many vegetarians still enjoy dairy foods. They offer a rich source of calcium, protein, zinc, and B12. Be careful when choosing yogurt, cheese, and cream, as these products can contain hidden animal-derived ingredients. Look out for rennet in cheese and gelatin in yogurt and cream. Read through the section on animal-derived ingredients (page 42) for more information.

Aim for around 0–2 servings/day. One serving equals one of the following:

- 1 cup milk or yogurt
- ½ cup cottage cheese, quark, or ricotta cheese
- Approximately 2 slices of cheese

The following are good nutrient-dense sources of dairy:

- Cheese (check for rennet and added preservatives)
- Milk
- Natural, whole-milk yogurt (with beneficial probiotics and no sugars, thickeners, or other additives)
- Quark

EGGS

Eggs offer a good source of protein, iron, zinc, and B12, and although not eaten by strict vegetarians, many vegetarians will include them in their diet. Always choose certified, free-range eggs and never battery-cage or barn-laid.

Aim for around 0–1 serving/day. One serving equals one whole egg.

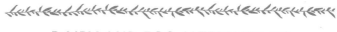

DAIRY AND EGG ALTERNATIVES

For strict vegetarians who avoid dairy and eggs, there are lots of store-brought or homemade alternatives that make great substitutes in your favorite meals. Choose soy, almond, oat, or rice milk—all the different brands available offer different flavors and consistencies. Try a variety until you find one you really like and look for those with no sugar or artificial additives for the healthiest choice. Nut and seed milks are easy to make at home, too; jump online for inspiration and recipes.

Soy yogurt, cheese, and cream cheese are readily available from natural foods stores and supermarkets. Alternatively, it's simple to make a great alternative to cream and yogurt in both savory and sweet dishes by soaking and grinding raw nuts like cashews and almonds. Cultured coconut yogurt is an excellent alternative to dairy yogurt as it contains all the beneficial probiotics found in natural yogurt. It's available from natural foods stores and some supermarkets, and you can also make your own at home.

If your diet is egg-free, look for soy or other egg-free mayonnaise alternatives and try one of the commercial egg substitutes or chia gel (see glossary) in baking and cooking.

VEGGIE PANTRY BASICS

Oils. There are two main types of oils to keep on hand—those for frying and cooking and those for use in dressings and sauces. For general frying, choose sunflower, rice bran, or peanut oil. To add the lovely flavor of olive oil to your dishes, add a little to your cooking oil in the pan. Save those full of flavor, like extra-virgin olive oil, plus nut and seed oils, such as sesame seed, macadamia, and walnut, for dressings and marinades.

Sauces and Vinegars. Sauces and vinegars are a great way to add extra flavor to the dishes you create. Be sure to check labels for animal-derived ingredients, especially in Asian-style sauces, which may contain fish or shellfish. Go for those sauces with little to no added sugar, salt, preservatives, and additives. Try tamari or soy sauce, kecap manis (dark soy sauce), harissa, sambal oelek, sweet chili sauce, tamarind paste, traditional curry pastes, and tomato paste. And look for things like apple cider vinegar, rice wine vinegar, raspberry vinegar, and balsamic vinegar for use in dressings and marinades.

Herbs. Where you can, choose fresh herbs or even better, have a go at growing your own. Look for fresh basil, parsley, cilantro, thyme, mint, and chives—perfect for adding their fresh and punchy flavors to nearly every type of meal. Use them by the handful in salads, pasta, and soups. Use the more pungent-flavored herbs, like sage, rosemary, tarragon, and dill, a little more sparingly in things like roasted vegetable dishes and rich, creamy sauces. When purchasing dried herbs, only buy a little at a time. They lose much of their flavor after just a short time on the shelf.

Spices. The world of spices is a world full of aromatic color and warm flavor. They can transform any dish into something truly special.

Experiment with different combinations and use them in nearly every type of food you prepare. Look for paprika, turmeric, cayenne pepper, mustard seeds, fennel seeds, cumin seeds, coriander seeds, curry powder, dried chilies, bay leaves, curry leaves, star anise, cinnamon sticks, and saffron—their flavors are essential to creating tasty meals. Freshly ground and roasted spices have the best flavor. Grind seeds and grains with a mortar and pestle before using, and either add them to your oil and fry over medium-low heat until fragrant before adding the rest of your ingredients, or sprinkle them over vegetables and toss with oil to coat before roasting. The aromatic flavor of spices will not last forever, so buy them a little at a time.

Nutrition-Boosting Foods. Take a trip down the aisle of your local health or natural foods store and you'll soon discover the wealth of nutrient-dense superfoods available. Look for raw cacao, spirulina, chlorella, hemp and chia seeds, nutritional yeast, blackstrap molasses, and natural protein powders made from yeast, whey, rice, and a variety of seeds. These are all powerful foods to include in your vegetarian diet, as they contain a host of important vitamins and minerals.

Although some can be expensive, you only need to use a little at a time and most, if not all, will keep well in either the fridge or pantry for a few months. Add spirulina, chlorella, protein, and cacao powders to smoothies and juices and cacao nibs plus hemp and chia seeds to your breakfast cereal. Blackstrap molasses is wonderful in both baked and savory dishes. Nutritional yeast has a lovely nutty flavor and is great sprinkled in a large variety of dishes for added flavor and nutrition.

While there is continuing research into the true "super" benefits of things like raw cacao, many agree they are an excellent addition to your diet. If you have any concerns, always speak to a professional nutritionist or doctor.

Fortified Foods. Fortified foods are processed foods with added vitamins and/or minerals. Look for nondairy milks such as soy, rice, oat, and almond fortified with things like calcium, protein, vitamin D, and vitamin B12. There are also fortified breakfast cereals available, often with added iron, calcium, and/or protein. These pre-packaged and readily available products come in a wide variety and are great for those who avoid dairy or are simply looking for a handy way to add extra nutrients to a vegetarian diet.

Avoiding Animal-Derived Ingredients

When buying processed food, it's worth taking a closer look at the label. There's a host of processed foods that contain ingredients made from meat and animal products—most commonly rennet in cheese; animal fat in spreadable butters, margarine, and frozen pastry; gelatin in processed yogurts, cream, and confections, packaged desserts, and icing on store-brought cakes.

Also keep an eye out for animal fat in fries, packaged cakes, cookies, and other bakery items; animal content in stocks/soups; and fish/shellfish in sauces and marinades. For many vegetarians, it can be important to avoid products that contain animal-derived ingredients. Check out the list below to learn more about these ingredients and how to avoid them in your vegetarian diet.

RENNET

Found in cheese, rennet is an enzyme traditionally made from the lining of calves' stomachs, and a good portion of the cheese available at your supermarket will contain this animal-derived ingredient. However, a growing number of cheese manufacturers now use a non-animal rennet. Look for cheese that clearly states "vegetarian" or "suitable for vegetarians" on the front. If in doubt, check the list of ingredients and choose those where the rennet or enzyme is identified as non-animal, vegetable, or microbial (enzymes derived from fungal or bacterial sources).

GELATIN

Gelatin is a by-product of the slaughterhouse industry and made from animal hides, hooves, bones, cartilage, and tendons. It's present in many processed foods and is often in low-fat yogurts, cream, jelly, confections, and ready-made desserts, to name but a few. There are vegetarian gelling agents such as agar and carrageenan that may be used by some manufacturers, so check the listed ingredients carefully on these kinds of products.

ANIMAL FAT (SUET/LARD)

Animal fat is the carcass fat from animals and again is a product of the slaughterhouse industry. It is often labeled as suet or lard and can be found in many frozen pastries, pre-packaged cakes, cookies, spreadable (softened) butters, and margarines. Another place to look out for lard is in fries, which may be fried in animal fat. Just ask in advance—there are many places that use vegetable oils instead.

FISH AND SHELLFISH–DERIVED INGREDIENTS

Some sauces, soups, dressings, and processed foods contain fish, or fish products. Most commonly these are Worcestershire sauce, Caesar salad dressings, and Asian-style sauces, dressings, and packaged soups. Keep an eye out for anchovies, crustaceans, fish sauce, and bonito or aspic, caviar, and chitin (made from crab shells) in the products you buy.

ANIMAL-CONTENT STOCKS

Some pre-packaged foods, especially soups, can contain animal-derived stock. Plus, always check the labels on the vegetable stock you buy; even some "vegetable stocks" will contain animal products. Look for vegetable-derived or no-animal-content stocks for your kitchen.

For Vegans

DAIRY

Dairy is present in a variety of common bakery items, including most conventional store-bought cakes, muffins, cookies, and some types of bread. Also look for dairy in popular sauces like hollandaise, creamy pasta sauces, dressings, and soups. Simply read labels carefully on the processed foods you buy, as many contain hidden dairy ingredients. Luckily, a growing number of products will now highlight dairy on the ingredient label, making it easy to quickly identify.

EGGS

Processed foods such as mayonnaise, dressings, and sauces, as well as bakery goods like cakes, some cookies, and desserts, will contain egg and egg-derived ingredients such as albumin. Look for egg-free alternatives like soy mayonnaise, and choose packaged foods carefully if you wish to avoid egg in the foods you eat.

Chapter 2

HOW TO BECOME A
HAPPY VEGGIE

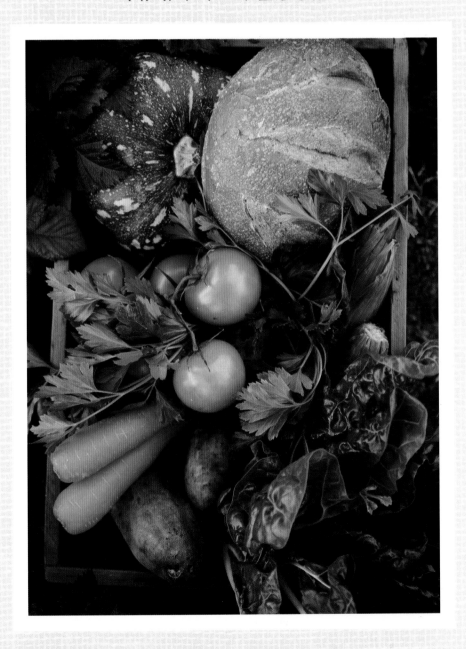

As a happy vegetarian, you'll feel fit, active, well nourished, and never like you're missing out on the things you love to eat. Keep in mind that being a happy veggie is all about enjoying the journey—the discovery of new ingredients and flavors and the positive effect conscious eating can have on your health and well-being. It can be a daunting prospect, making the switch to a plant-based diet, and for many, knowing where to start and how to keep motivated are probably the biggest hurdles. Yet the choice to be vegetarian doesn't have to be difficult.

Get excited and inspired by the wealth of wholesome and tasty foods available, and look to your own ideals for motivation and encouragement. It's these things that allow you to stay positive and feel good about the choices you're making. Enjoying the veggie food on your plate and having fun creating tasty meat-free meals mean you never feel like you're missing out on the things you love to eat, just as having a strong conviction behind your choice to be meat-free means you're far more likely to stay committed and positive about the change.

Slowly building a knowledge and love of healthy vegetarian foods into your diet is by far the simplest and most effective approach to being a happy veggie. The following are some great ideas on how to get started and stay motivated, with a few hints and tips on having a little fun along the way.

Start with one meat-free day a week. Swapping your usual dinner for a vegetarian meal just one day a week can be a good starting point for those who want to take it slow or are completely unfamiliar with vegetarian food. It's only one day a week, so no pressure to make a complete overnight change in your diet. Plus it's a fun and relaxed way for the whole family to get on board and learn about the different types of delicious vegetarian foods there are to be had.

Replace one meat product (animal) at a time. Start by cutting out only one type of meat—maybe from an animal whose welfare most concerns you, such as pigs or chickens. Tempeh, tofu, and faux-meats make a great starting point for those who still want to eat something familiar but are looking for a vegetarian alternative. Try tofu or tempeh in place of chicken and one of the many varieties of veggie sausages instead of your typical pork or beef sausage, and go from there.

Re-create your favorite meals. Discover just how easy and fun it is creating a vegetarian version of your favorite meals by substituting beans, lentils, grains, tofu, and other soy products for the meat. Get creative with lots of herbs, spices, dried fruits, nuts, and seeds, and enjoy the process. Realizing your favorite meals can be just as or even more delicious transformed into a vegetarian alternative is one of the best ways to kick-start being a happy veggie.

Get your family and friends on board. Discuss the reasons behind your choice with your family and friends, and encourage them to get on board and try more veggie foods, too. Making the change with someone else is a great idea, and having the support and encouragement of those around you makes all the difference. Plus it's fun and helpful having someone else to compare vegetarian foods and share recipes with.

Enjoy the journey. Be mindful of the positive impact a vegetarian diet can have. If you ever feel discouraged or uninspired, take a moment to remind yourself of all the good things that can come from your choice to be vegetarian. You're choosing healthy, wholesome foods that are good for your body, and you're making a conscious effort to do something positive not only for yourself but for the lives of animals. Staying true to your convictions and reminding yourself of the reasons behind your own choice to be vegetarian will help you stay positive and motivated along the way.

Get inspired. Seek out lots of inspiration for mouthwatering vegetarian meals. Food inspiration is available everywhere—online and in bookstores, libraries, and magazines. Start following veggie blogs, raid your library for veggie cookbooks, and have some fun in the kitchen cooking up a huge variety of tasty and inspiring meals. You'll learn more about vegetarian food, cooking techniques, and ingredients, plus discover just how varied and exciting the world of vegetarian food can be.

Become part of the community. There's a rich and diverse world of vegetarians out there. For lots of great support, friendship, ideas, and motivation, consider joining a vegetarian society. Log onto web communities like your local Meatless Monday campaign or one of the many active vegetarian forums. Sharing your experiences and learning from others is a fantastic step to becoming a happy veggie.

Share the joy. Go all out and invite your family and friends around for a veggie feast—it will get you cooking with new and exciting ingredients and sharing with others the abundant and delicious world of vegetarian food. It's a fun and positive way to bring the joys of food and being veggie to those you love.

Out and About

Being a vegetarian doesn't have to be an issue—check out the following tips on navigating a meat-eating world with ease.

Eating out. Go for Japanese, Indian, Tibetan, or Mexican cuisine, as you're bound to find a few great veggie options, or jump online and check out one of the many sites offering information on popular vegetarian-friendly restaurants in your neighborhood. If your friends or family are choosing the restaurant, make sure they're aware you're vegetarian so you don't end up in a steak house.

Although many restaurants will offer at least one vegetarian option, it may not always be vegan. Don't be afraid to request a special meal or ask to have one ingredient or another removed or replaced from a dish on the menu. Or, try calling the restaurant in advance to make sure you'll have a suitable vegetarian option available.

Holidays, parties, or special occasions. Always let your hosts know in advance that you're vegetarian to avoid any embarrassment, or worse, offense. The very best idea is the offer to bring a dish or two yourself—a win-win situation, as your host doesn't have to stress over preparing what may be an unfamiliar meat-free option and you get to share with others all the veggie foods you love. Check out the recipes starting on page 77 for ideas on great vegetarian meals to prepare for holidays and special occasions so no one feels like they're missing out on traditional fare.

Traveling. Many airlines now offer a vegan choice for their in-flight meals. Even better, pack your own vegetarian option to be sure you're getting tasty and nutritious food. Things like nuts, seeds, dried fruits, cereal bars, sandwiches, salads, and some fresh fruits and vegetables make great traveling snacks on long drives or flights. When in a different country, make sure to do some research on finding vegetarian options before leaving. Once you arrive, stock up at the local store on things like bottled water, fresh fruit, and healthy vegetarian snacks to keep with you as you travel around.

When people question your choice. There will always be those few who want to challenge your decision to be vegetarian—just as there will always be those who feel the need to challenge anything they find unfamiliar. Don't take it personally; be kind and stay positive when dealing with others' negative reactions. The very best thing to do is invite them over for a delicious vegetarian meal or suggest places online or in books where they can discover for themselves more about factory farming and/or vegetarian nutrition.

While it can be difficult dealing with the negative reactions of those close to you, remind yourself of the reason you made the choice, and stay focused on becoming a happy and healthy veggie. Your positive approach, glowing good health, and happiness are the very best advocates for becoming a vegetarian.

What to Eat When You Feel Like Something Familiar

Eating food that is familiar as well as tasty and satisfying is easy on a vegetarian diet, and transforming a traditional meat dish into something completely vegetarian can be quite simple, with a little creativity. The following table is a quick reference guide to replacing animal products with plant-based alternatives. You'll also find recipe suggestions from the book to help you on your way.

As a great starting point, try re-creating some of your favorite recipes, switching out the meat for the vegetarian alternatives offered below. You'll soon discover the joy and satisfaction of transforming a dish you love into a vegetarian masterpiece.

MAKE THE SWITCH		
Beef	▷	Lentils or mushrooms
Lamb	▷	Chickpeas, eggplant, or potatoes
Chicken, fish, and shellfish	▷	Tempeh or tofu
Diced bacon	▷	Pine nuts
Anchovies	▷	Salted capers
Cream	▷	Soaked and ground almonds or cashew nuts
Eggs in baking	▷	Chia gel

Another easy option, especially for new vegetarians, is to try some of the many vegetarian "meats" (often made from soy products but also from vegetables, beans, and lentils) now available in most supermarkets. There is a huge variety of ready-made vegetarian burgers, sausages, and faux-meats to purchase—look for those that are minimally processed and contain predominately natural ingredients. Products like these make it easy to switch out the meat for a vegetarian alternative in nearly any meal you can think of.

Try these recipes for a veggie take on something familiar:

GROUND BEEF
Lentil Bolognese Lasagna (page 145)
Mushroom Cannelloni with Cauliflower Béchamel (page 115)
Red Lentil Sausage Rolls (page 164)
Dal Kofta Balls and Curry (page 125)
Spicy Lentil Tart with Pomegranate and Mint (page 182)

SAUSAGES, STEAK, AND BURGERS

Buckwheat, Mushroom, Rye Burger with Quick
Tomato Relish and Kale Chips (page 142)

Grilled Mushrooms on Rye with Fresh Tomato Salsa
and Creamy Horseradish Sauce (page 99)

Fragrant Couscous with Veg Sausage, Chickpeas,
Almonds, and Apricots (page 137)

CHICKEN

Tempeh Pot Pies (page 140)

Satay Tempeh Lettuce Wraps (page 104)

Sweet Potato and Kale Quesadilla (page 151)

Barbecued Piri Piri Pumpkin and Tofu Skewers with
Date and Walnut Couscous (page 171)

FISH & SHELLFISH

Soda-Battered Eggplant with Carrot Chips, Sprout
Salad, and Fresh Pickle (page 133)

Tofu Tacos with Slaw, Grilled Corn, Chili Cashew
Cream, and Roasted Salsa (page 157)

Soy and Szechuan Pepper Tofu with Wasabi Pea Puree (page 161)

Chapter 3

30-DAY VEGETARIAN MEAL GUIDE

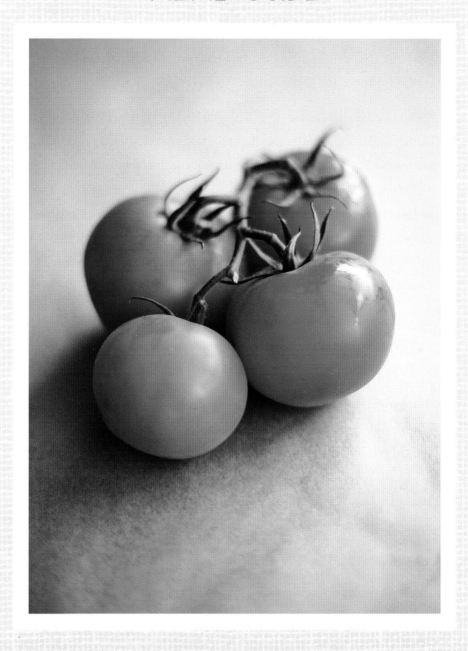

The following is a flexible guide to help you gradually adopt new vegetarian foods and recipes into your everyday diet. Over the course of the 30 days you will work your way through a bounty of tasty vegetarian recipes and nutritious plant-based ingredients. (The recipes listed can be found in the recipe section, as indicated, while some of the simpler, do-it-yourself suggestions do not include a corresponding recipe.) All the recipes in the book are rated with a difficulty level. One-star recipes are super-easy, two stars mean a little extra preparation is required, and three-star recipes have a few trickier techniques.

It's an introduction to eating as a vegetarian and starts with swapping just a few of your regular meals throughout the day for a vegetarian alternative and adopting only one or two completely meat-free days a week. Each week you can chooses to adopt more vegetarian meals, or just try some of the veggie recipes with suggested meat accompaniments, if you prefer. When the choice is left up to you, it's your call whether you eat vegetarian or not, making it easy to adapt at your own pace.

If you want to take it slow, stick to the first week's guidelines for a couple of extra weeks until you feel ready to move on. If you're feeling ready to go completely vegetarian, skip to week four and give it a try.

By no means a strict diet to follow or a calculated nutritional plan, this is more a general guide to eating a healthy vegetarian diet. Change, add, or adapt the meal suggestions to your needs, and look to this guide for inspiration and ideas to help you adopt lots of interesting and delicious vegetarian foods into your everyday diet.

An Overview of the 30-Day Plan

WEEK ONE

Try 1–2 vegetarian meals each day. Aim for 1–2 meat-free days this week. (On one of the meat-free days, you decide whether to eat vegetarian or try the recipe accompanied by meat.)

WEEK TWO

Try 2 vegetarian meals each day. Aim for 2–3 meat-free days this week. (On one of the meat-free days, you decide whether to eat vegetarian or try the recipe accompanied by meat.)

WEEK THREE

Try 2–3 vegetarian meals each day. Aim for 3–5 meat-free days this week. (On two of the meat-free days, you decide whether to eat vegetarian or try the recipes accompanied by meat.)

WEEK FOUR

Try 3 vegetarian meals each day. Aim for 5–7 meat-free days this week. (On two of the meat-free days, you decide whether to eat vegetarian or try the recipes accompanied by meat.)

WEEK FIVE: THE LAST TWO DAYS

Try 3 vegetarian meals each day. Aim for meat-free every day this week.

TIPS Feel free to include a dessert on any day of the week. Just be sure to check for hidden animal-derived ingredients like gelatin and animal fat if you choose processed items such as ice cream or pre-packaged cakes, sweets, and desserts.

THE 30-DAY PLAN

Try 1–2 vegetarian meals each day. Aim for 1–2 meat-free days this week. All vegetarian meals are labeled with Ⓥ.

Day 1

MONDAY Go for Meat-Free Today

BREAKFAST	Toasted Multigrain Granola (page 88) with soy milk and fresh fruit Ⓥ Breakfast Smoothie (page 86)
LUNCH	Whole-grain wrap with vegetarian sausage, grated raw vegetables, sprouts, and hummus Ⓥ
DINNER	Lentil Bolognese Lasagna (page 145) + green salad or steamed greens Ⓥ
SNACK	1 peach + a few raw Brazil nuts Ⓥ

Day 2

TUESDAY

BREAKFAST	Coco Banana Overnight Oats (page 84) topped with fresh fruit Ⓥ Fresh fruit and vegetable juice
LUNCH	Your favorite lunch
DINNER	Your regular dinner
SNACK	Raw vegetable sticks with hummus Ⓥ

Day 3

WEDNESDAY

BREAKFAST	Whole-grain toast with grilled mushrooms and hummus Ⓥ Fruit Smoothie (page 74)
LUNCH	Your regular lunch
DINNER	Your favorite dinner
SNACK	2 rice cakes with Walnut Paste (page 81) and sprouts Ⓥ

Day 4
THURSDAY

BREAKFAST	Coco Banana Overnight Oats (page 84) topped with soy yogurt and fresh fruit **Ⓥ** Fresh fruit and vegetable juice
LUNCH	Soba noodles with leafy greens, marinated tofu, pickled ginger, sesame seeds, and tamari **Ⓥ** *(Option: Add your choice of responsibly caught salmon or tuna.)*
DINNER	Your regular dinner
SNACK	1 slice of Seeded Banana Bread with Dried Figs and Turkish Apricots (page 92) **Ⓥ**

Day 5
FRIDAY

BREAKFAST	Dark rye toast with avocado and a sprinkle of hemp or chia seeds **Ⓥ** Green Smoothie (page 75)
LUNCH	Protein-Packed Salad (page 69) + multigrain crackers **Ⓥ** *(Option: Add your choice of certified free-range meat to the salad.)*
DINNER	Your regular dinner
SNACK	Miso soup **Ⓥ**

Day 6
SATURDAY Go for Meat-Free Today

BREAKFAST	Toasted Multigrain Granola (page 88) with soy milk, coconut yogurt, and fresh fruit
LUNCH	Sweet Potato and Kale Quesadillas (page 151) Sprout Salad (page 133)
DINNER	Dal Kofta Curry (page 125) **Ⓥ** *(Option: Serve the above recipe accompanied by your favorite meat-based curry made from preferably certified free-range meat of your choice.)*
SNACK	1 Whole-Grain Cacao Chip Cookie (page 94) **Ⓥ** Soy yogurt

Day 7
SUNDAY

BREAKFAST	Whole Wheat/Spelt Pancakes (page 90) with fresh fruit and nut butter **Ⓥ** Fresh fruit and vegetable juice
LUNCH	Heirloom Tomato and Onion Jam Tart with Thyme, Olive Oil, Buckwheat Crust (page 174) + green salad **Ⓥ**
DINNER	Your favorite dinner
SNACK	1 orange + a handful of Toasted Multigrain Granola (page 88) **Ⓥ**

Try 2 vegetarian meals each day. Aim for 2–3 meat-free days this week.

Day 8

MONDAY Go for Meat-Free Today

BREAKFAST	Coco Banana Overnight Oats (page 84) with stewed fruit ⓥ Green Smoothie (page 75)
LUNCH	Protein-Packed Salad (page 69) ⓥ Fresh fruit and vegetable juice
DINNER	Pita Pockets with Carrot Falafel and Creamy Harissa Sauce (page 97) ⓥ
SNACK	½ banana, 1 dried fig, and 2 walnuts ⓥ

Day 9

TUESDAY

BREAKFAST	Toasted Multigrain Granola (page 88) with soy milk and fresh fruit ⓥ Breakfast Smoothie (page 86)
LUNCH	Whole-grain wrap with greens, grated vegetables, chickpeas, cashews, and tahini ⓥ Fresh vegetable juice
DINNER	Your choice of dinner
SNACK	1 slice of Seeded Banana Bread with Dried Figs and Turkish Apricots (page 92) ⓥ

Day 10

WEDNESDAY Go for Meat-Free Today

BREAKFAST	Toasted whole-grain muffin with almond butter, sliced fresh figs or banana, and maple syrup ⓥ Fresh fruit and vegetable juice
LUNCH	Protein-Packed Salad (page 69) + multigrain crackers ⓥ Soy yogurt
DINNER	Roasted Pumpkin and Sage Spelt Pasta with Pumpkin Seed and Spinach Pesto (page 154) *(Option: Try the above recipe served with a side of preferably certified free-range beef or lamb.)*
SNACK	Green Smoothie (page 75) ⓥ 1 Whole-Grain Cacao Chip Cookie (page 94)

Day 11

THURSDAY

BREAKFAST	Dark rye toast with baked beans and avocado ⓥ Fruit Smoothie (page 74)
LUNCH	Corn tortillas with cooked or canned red beans, avocado, grated carrot, and soy cheese ⓥ
DINNER	Your choice of dinner
SNACK	Handful of fresh berries + a few raw pistachios or Brazil nuts ⓥ Fresh vegetable juice

Day 12

FRIDAY

BREAKFAST	Toasted Multigrain Granola (page 88) with almond milk and fresh fruit ⓥ Fresh fruit and vegetable juice
LUNCH	Rye bread sandwich with grilled tempeh, grated raw veg, sprouts, and tahini ⓥ
DINNER	Your choice of dinner
SNACK	Wedges of green apple spread with nut butter and sprinkled with chia seeds ⓥ

Day 13

SATURDAY Go For Meat-Free Today

BREAKFAST	Whole-grain pita with grilled mushrooms, arugula, and hummus ⓥ Fresh fruit and vegetable juice
LUNCH	Red Lentil Sausage Rolls (page 164) ⓥ Shaved Fennel and Green Apple Salad with Roasted Grapes and Hazelnuts (page 180)
DINNER	Trio of Pizzas (page 167) ⓥ
SNACK	1 peach + a few raw Brazil nuts ⓥ

Day 14

SUNDAY

BREAKFAST	Coco Banana Overnight Oats (page 84) with nut butter ⓥ Fresh fruit and vegetable juice
LUNCH	Your favorite lunch
DINNER	Buckwheat, Mushroom, Rye Burgers with Quick Tomato Relish and Kale Chips (page 142) ⓥ
SNACK	Raw vegetable sticks and rice crackers with Tofu-tzatziki (page 82) ⓥ

Try 2–3 vegetarian meals each day. Aim for 3–5 meat-free days this week.

Day 15
MONDAY Go for Meat-Free Today

BREAKFAST	Coco Banana Overnight Oats (page 84) with fresh fruit and nut butter ⓥ Green Smoothie (page 75)
LUNCH	Protein-Packed Salad (page 69) ⓥ + whole-grain muffin spread with Kale Pesto (page 81)
DINNER	Curried Black Rice Soup with Green Veg and Silken Tofu (page 130) ⓥ
SNACK	1 orange + a handful of Toasted Multigrain Granola (page 88) ⓥ

Day 16
TUESDAY Go for Meat-Free Today

BREAKFAST	Toasted Multigrain Granola (page 88) with almond milk and fresh fruit ⓥ Fresh vegetable juice
LUNCH	Soba noodles with leafy greens, marinated tofu, pickled ginger, sesame seeds, and tamari ⓥ
DINNER	Barbecued Piri Piri Pumpkin and Tofu Skewers with Date and Walnut Couscous (page 171) ⓥ *(Option: If you prefer, try the recipe above adding certified free-range chicken pieces along with, or instead of, the tofu.)*
SNACK	Seeded Banana Bread with Dried Figs and Turkish Apricots (page 92) ⓥ

Day 17
WEDNESDAY

BREAKFAST	Rye toast with avocado, grilled cherry tomatoes, and a drizzle of tahini ⓥ Breakfast Smoothie (page 86)
LUNCH	Protein-Packed Salad (page 69) ⓥ Fresh fruit and vegetable juice
DINNER	Your favorite dinner
SNACK	1 Whole-Grain Cacao Chip Cookie (page 94) ⓥ Green Smoothie (page 75)

Day 18

THURSDAY Go for Meat-Free Today

BREAKFAST	Coco Banana Overnight Oats (page 84) with fresh fruit and nut butter (V)
LUNCH	Whole-grain wrap with chickpeas, grated raw veg, sprouts, and tahini (V) Vegetable juice
DINNER	Fragrant Brown Rice and Puy Lentils with Grilled Vegetables and Pine Nut Cream (page 119) (V) *(Option: Serve the above recipe accompanied with preferably certified free-range lamb or beef.)*
SNACK	Raw vegetable sticks and rice crackers with Tofu-tzatziki (page 82) (V)

Day 19

FRIDAY Go for Meat-Free Today

BREAKFAST	Toasted Multigrain Granola (page 88) with soy milk and fresh fruit (V) Fresh fruit and vegetable juice
LUNCH	Soba Noodles and Sesame-Ginger Greens with Shiitake-Miso Broth (page 107) (V)
DINNER	Soda-Battered Eggplant with Carrot Chips, Sprout Salad, and Fresh Pickle (page 133) (V)
SNACK	1 Whole-Grain Cacao Chip Cookie (page 94) (V) Soy yogurt

Day 20

SATURDAY Go for Meat-Free Today

BREAKFAST	Whole-grain toasted muffins with grilled tomatoes, baby spinach, and avocado (V) Breakfast Smoothie (page 86)
LUNCH	Soy and Szechuan Pepper Tofu with Wasabi Pea Puree (page 161) + a side of brown rice (V)
DINNER	Mushroom Cannelloni with Cauliflower Béchamel (page 115) + steamed greens (V)
SNACK	1 kiwifruit + a small handful of Toasted Multigrain Granola (page 88) (V)

Day 21

SUNDAY

BREAKFAST	Whole Wheat/Spelt Pancakes (page 90) with stewed fruit and coconut yogurt (V)
LUNCH	Warm Vegetable and Barley Salad with Orange, Honey, and Thyme Dressing (page 110) (V)
DINNER	Your favorite Sunday night dinner
SNACK	Raw vegetable sticks with hummus (V)

Try 3 vegetarian meals each day. Aim for 5–7 meat-free days this week.

Day 22
MONDAY

BREAKFAST	Coco Banana Overnight Oats (page 84) with fresh fruit ⓥ Breakfast Smoothie (page 86)
LUNCH	Super Beet Soup with Apple, Celery, and Turmeric (page 103) + rye bread ⓥ
DINNER	Fragrant Couscous with Veg Sausage, Chickpeas, Almonds, and Apricots (page 137) + steamed greens ⓥ
SNACK	2 corn cakes with Kale Pesto (page 81), cherry tomatoes, and sprouts ⓥ

Day 23
TUESDAY Go for Meat-Free Today

BREAKFAST	Toasted whole-grain muffin with almond butter, sliced fresh figs or banana, and maple syrup ⓥ Vegetable juice
LUNCH	Protein-Packed Salad (page 69) ⓥ Soy yogurt
DINNER	Curried Lentil Soup with Coconut and Cashews (page 148) ⓥ
SNACK	Handful of fresh berries + a few raw pistachios or Brazil nuts ⓥ

Day 24
WEDNESDAY Go for Meat-Free Today

BREAKFAST	Toasted Multigrain Granola (page 88) with soy milk and stewed fruit ⓥ
LUNCH	Steamed brown rice bowl with grated vegetables, marinated tofu, avocado, sesame seeds, and tamari ⓥ
DINNER	Grilled Mushrooms on Rye with Fresh Tomato Salsa and Creamy Horseradish Sauce (page 99) ⓥ
SNACK	Green Smoothie (page 75) + a few multigrain crackers ⓥ

Day 25
THURSDAY Go for Meat-Free Today

BREAKFAST	Rye toast with tahini and sliced banana + maple syrup and chia seeds ⓥ Breakfast Smoothie (page 86)
LUNCH	Protein-Packed Salad (page 69) ⓥ Fresh fruit and vegetable juice
DINNER	Baked Fennel and Vegetable Medley with Quinoa (page 128) ⓥ *(Option: Serve the above with responsibly caught grilled fish.)*
SNACK	1 Whole-Grain Cacao Chip Cookie (page 94) ⓥ 1 orange

Day 26

FRIDAY Go for Meat-Free Today

BREAKFAST	Toasted Multigrain Granola (page 88) with fresh fruit ⓥ Green Smoothie (page 75)
LUNCH	Protein-Packed Salad (page 69) ⓥ + whole-grain muffin spread with avocado Vegetable juice
DINNER	Tofu Tacos with Slaw, Grilled Corn, Chili Cashew Cream, and Roasted Salsa (page 157) ⓥ *(Option: Replace some or all of the tofu in the above recipe with responsibly caught fish.)*
SNACK	Edamame, raw vegetable sticks, and rice crackers ⓥ

Day 27

SATURDAY Go for Meat-Free Today

BREAKFAST	Coco Banana Overnight Oats (page 84) with nut butter ⓥ
LUNCH	Satay Tempeh Lettuce Wraps (page 104) ⓥ
DINNER	Spicy Lentil Tart with Pomegranate and Mint (page 182) ⓥ Date and Walnut Couscous (page 171) + side of leafy greens
SNACK	Sliced banana and dried figs with sunflower and pumpkin seeds, drizzled with a little honey (or agave nectar) and a pinch of cinnamon ⓥ

Day 28

SUNDAY Go for Meat-Free Today

BREAKFAST	Dark rye toast with grilled mushrooms and Kale Pesto (page 81) ⓥ Fresh fruit and vegetable juice
LUNCH	Crispy Fried Polenta with Baby Kale and Sundried Tomatoes (page 177) ⓥ
DINNER	Tempeh Pot Pies (page 140) ⓥ
SNACK	Multigrain crackers ⓥ Green Smoothie (page 75)

Aim for meat-free every day.

Day 29
MONDAY Meat-Free

BREAKFAST	Toasted Multigrain Granola (page 88) with soy milk and fresh fruit (V)
LUNCH	Rye bread sandwich with vegetarian burger, grated raw veg, sprouts, and tahini (V)
DINNER	Baked Risotto with Tossed Green Vegetables (page 122) (V)
SNACK	Small handful of fresh berries + a few pistachios (V)

Day 30
TUESDAY Meat-Free

BREAKFAST	Coco Banana Overnight Oats (page 84) with fresh fruit + nut butter (V)
LUNCH	Protein-Packed Salad (page 69) Vegetable juice (V)
DINNER	Roasted Eggplant and Almond Pesto with Whole wheat Pasta (page 113) (V)
SNACK	1 Whole-Grain Cacao Chip Cookie (page 94) Green Smoothie (page 75) (V)

You made it! You've reached the end of your 30-day vegetarian transformation and the real journey has only just begun. By now you've hopefully sampled a wealth of delicious meat-free meals and discovered lots of tasty, nutrient-rich foods and ingredients that will inspire you to continue along your way to becoming a truly healthy and happy vegetarian for life!

Tips for Eating Veggie Every Day

Enjoying a diet packed with satisfying and nutritious meat-free meals is, ultimately, what will enable you to become a lifelong vegetarian. This chapter is full of inspiration for preparing meals you'll love to eat, nutritious foods for your family that will keep them coming back for more, and quick and simple snacks to feed hungry bellies on the go.

Included is information on breakfast, lunch, and dinner, with healthy snack ideas, plus smoothies and juices—all designed to help you build your complete vegetarian diet, full of delicious and satisfying foods and with all the vital nutrition and energy to thrive.

BREAKFAST

It's often called the most important meal of the day, and for good reason. A healthy breakfast will lift energy levels, ignite mental concentration, and boost metabolism. Kick-starting your day with a healthy breakfast will help you to feel active, fit, and healthy.

While it can be one of the busiest times of the day, especially if you're off to work early or getting kids ready for school, taking the time to enjoy a healthy breakfast is important. Fortunately, breakfast foods are some of the most nutritious and delicious, with a bounty of essential vitamins and minerals on offer from fresh fruits, cereals, whole-grains, nuts, and seeds.

If you're running around in the morning getting ready for your day, try some of the following ideas to take the pressure off preparing a nutritious and tasty breakfast for you and your family.

Throughout the year, buy bulk seasonal fruits for freezing and preserving. Things like mangos, bananas, and berries freeze well.

Simply chop them into slices or cubes and freeze in bags or containers, perfect for a quick smoothie in the morning. Berries, apples, pears, and stone fruit are all ideal for making stewed fruit, which is a delicious and quick addition to your granola or oatmeal. To stew most fruits, simply chop and add to a pan with enough water to cover the bottom and brown sugar or maple syrup to taste. Simmer gently until the fruit is soft and gooey. Store in jars for a few days in the fridge or freeze in small portions, defrosting overnight in the fridge.

Overnight oats are the ultimate healthy breakfast solution for the time-poor. Easily prepared the night before—simply combine all the ingredients together and pop in the fridge. In the morning you have an instant, ready-to-eat, healthy breakfast. You can prepare the oats in jars or containers, making them portable for a delicious and nutritious breakfast on the go. Check out the recipe on page 84 and get creative by adding you favorite fruits, nuts, and seeds.

Breakfast smoothies. As a nutritious, simple, and speedy breakfast, smoothies make a great choice for busy people. A handy tip is to cut up lots of fruit in advance and freeze separate smoothie "packs" in your freezer with a combination of fruits ready to blend for a single smoothie serving. Add things like rice or seed protein powders and/or nut butters for extra protein. It'll kick-start your metabolism and keep you powering through the day. Check out the recipe or the handy "Build a Fruit Smoothie" chart on page 74 for loads of inspiration.

Choose whole-grain cereals and granola. Make your own ahead of time or choose from the large variety available at your natural foods store and supermarket. Look for those packed with lots of different grains, cereals, seeds, and nuts, and without added sugar for the healthiest option. Store a selection in different large jars in the pantry to contend with fussy eaters. Top with fresh or stewed fruit, soy, oat, almond, or rice milk, and things like sunflower, pumpkin, hemp, or chia seeds. Alternatively, look for store-bought seed-and-nut combinations for a quick sprinkle of added nutrition on top.

Feel like toast? Choose whole-grain, multigrain, or rye breads and top with nut butters and sliced fresh or dried fruits. Almond butter and sliced banana with a little maple syrup is good, or try tahini with dried figs and honey or maple syrup. For something savory, go for avocado and sliced cherry tomatoes with fresh sprouts, or fried mushrooms with arugula and cracked pepper.

Smoothies, toast, oatmeal, and granola are all quick and nutritious breakfast options—with a variety of ways to add lots of extra goodness and flavor. Check out the recipes chapter for some inspiration for creating fuss-free and healthy breakfasts the whole family will enjoy. You'll also find a couple of more extravagant recipes for those weekend mornings when you feel like something a little special.

LUNCH

At lunchtime, go for fresh and wholesome foods to fill the gap and power you through the rest of the day. Whole-grains, legumes, and soy products are great to keep you feeling full and sustain your energy. When at home or for a special occasion, take the time to prepare a nutritious meal like those found in the "Lighter Meals" recipe section that starts on page 97.

Alternatively, for a speedy lunch at home or a healthy packed lunch solution, salads and sandwiches or wraps are the obvious choice. They're both portable and provide lots of opportunity for added goodness and flavor. Check out the following ideas for some healthy inspiration.

Sandwiches and wraps make a great packed lunch. Go for whole wheat, rye, or seeded buns and bread, rice, or barley wraps, corn tortillas, and whole wheat pita pocket breads. Load them up with fresh grated vegetables, sprouts, and leafy greens. Add things like chickpeas, beans, sliced firm plain or seasoned tofu, veggie sausages, and burgers or hummus and tahini for more protein.

Prepare ingredients in advance for a quick and healthy addition to salads. Rice, quinoa, buckwheat, and barley can be cooked ahead of time and stored in the fridge for a few days and are a quick and nutritious addition to salads. Or, cook a few veggie sausages the night before to add to your salad the next day. Plus, things like canned beans, lentils, and firm, ready-marinated or seasoned tofu require no cooking and are a great quick-and-easy solution. Check out the handy "Build a Protein-Packed Salad" chart on page 69 for lots of healthy inspiration. Just be sure to dress the salad right before eating—a dressed and packed salad will quickly wilt.

Noodles make a great quick-and-nutritious lunch. Go for soba, ramen, or udon (which take only 4 minutes or so to cook). Toss the prepared noodles with things like leafy greens, broccoli, edamame, sprouts, green beans, tofu, pickled ginger, sliced avocado, or cold roasted vegetables, and dress with sesame oil or tahini and a little lime or lemon juice.

Don't forget your leftovers. Lots of meals make excellent leftovers for lunch. Cold roasted vegetable dishes are great simply reheated, or try adding them to a wrap or pocket bread with a tahini dressing and some fresh greens like arugula, baby spinach, or kale. Leftover pasta often reheats well, and dishes like curries and soups are even better when eaten the next day.

For healthy take-out options, think fresh and wholesome. Try to avoid overly processed, packaged foods and high-fat options like pastries, pies, and cheesy toasted sandwiches on a daily basis. Vegetarian cafes offering rice dishes, curries, and fresh salads are great for a quick meal. Or go for sandwiches and salads that offer added nutrition with whole-grain, fresh, and protein-packed ingredients.

BUILD A PROTEIN-PACKED SALAD		
	LEGUME	SOY
CHOOSE YOUR PROTEIN	Butter beans Chickpeas Kidney beans Lentils (cooked or canned)	Crumbed grilled tempeh Faux-meat Sliced cooked veggie sausage Tofu, cubed (seasoned or plain)
ADD GRAINS	Barley Bulgur Buckwheat Couscous	Millet Quinoa Rice
ADD GREENS	Arugula Beet greens Butter lettuce Kale	Romaine Spinach Sprouts Watercress
ADD CRUNCH	Apple Bell peppers Broccoli (raw) Carrot Celery	Cucumber Edamame Green beans Snow peas
TOP IT OFF	Almonds Cashews Hemp seeds Pecans	Sesame seeds Sunflower seeds Pumpkin seeds Walnuts
SOMETHING A LITTLE DIFFERENT	Dried apricots Dried cranberries	Dried figs Golden raisins
DRESS IT UP	Choose from the dressing recipes on page 78.	

DINNER

Whether it's a big fancy dinner or something simple and nutritious, there's nothing like a home-cooked meal to end the day. Look to the recipe section of this book for lots of inspiration. It's full of delicious and satisfying meals, including wholesome family dinners, simple nutritious meals, and lovely dishes for special occasions. During those busy weeknights when time is short, try some of the following tips to take the pressure off preparing hearty, nutritious dinners you'll love to eat with your family.

Look to some of the lunch suggestions starting on page 67. Hearty salads and quick noodle dishes also work well as simple dinner solutions.

Investing in a slow cooker or rice cooker can be a fantastic idea for the time-poor. Perfect for preparing anything like grains, rice, and even casseroles and soups in advance.

Roasted vegetables are simple to prepare, taste amazing, and provide lots of important vitamins and minerals. Simply preheat the oven, throw any chopped vegetables in a baking tray, drizzle with oil, add a few good pinches of your favorite herbs and spices (things like paprika, cumin seeds, cinnamon, thyme, and rosemary all work well), and toss to coat with a little pinch of salt flakes and cracked pepper. Bake the veggies in a 350°F oven for around 35–50 minutes (depending on which vegetables you used and your oven) until golden. Serve with any grain you like and bulk them out with a can of chickpeas or kidney beans, dress with some dried fruits, nuts, and seeds, or toss with fresh, leafy greens like baby spinach or cress.

Couscous is a fantastic, filling, and quick-to-prepare staple. Simply combine equal parts instant couscous and boiling water or vegetable stock, cover, and set aside for a few minutes. Once the liquid's absorbed, fluff with a fork, adding a little olive oil to help separate the grains. Serve warm or cold—add things like canned or cooked beans, chickpeas, or lentils, fresh herbs like parsley, mint, or basil, plus dried fruits, nuts, seeds, and diced fruits and vegetables like tomato, carrot, cucumber, celery, apple, or peach. Get inventive and create your own combination of favorite flavors and textures.

When you really don't feel like cooking. Don't look past humble baked beans on toast. Go for low-salt and -sugar varieties and choose healthy whole-grain or seeded breads. Or try breakfast for dinner— things like granola or a warm bowl of oatmeal, loaded with fresh or dried fruits, nuts, seeds, and maybe some coconut or dairy yogurt can be a filling and healthy meal when you don't feel like getting out the pots and pans.

SNACKS

Enjoying a healthy snack can be a great way to maintain your energy levels throughout the day—plus boost your intake of important vitamins and minerals. Sticking to a small portion and keeping it healthy is the key. A pantry and fridge well stocked with lots of nutritious snacking options means you've always got a variety of healthy foods to choose from when hunger strikes.

When out and about, a great idea is to make your own snacks and take them with you or stash some healthy options in your desk drawer at work. Check out the following for some quick ideas, plus the banana bread recipe (page 92), cookie recipe (page 94), or the Tofu-tzatziki (page 82) for healthy and delicious snacks to keep your body and belly happy.

Fruit, nut, and seed combos. Try some of the following or create your own using your favorite fruits, dried fruits, nuts, seeds, and nut or seed butters.

- Slices of green apple spread with almond butter and sprinkled with chia seeds
- A small bowl of sliced banana and dried figs, sunflower seeds, and pumpkin seeds, drizzled with a little tahini and honey, and topped with a pinch of cinnamon
- A handful of seed and nut granola with a sliced orange
- A small handful of fresh blueberries with a few raw pistachio nuts
- One kiwifruit and a couple of raw Brazil nuts and sunflower seeds

Combinations like these are packed with vital essential nutrients and are a good source of energy to help you get through the day.

Raw veggies are another great option. Go for edamame, carrot, cucumber, bell pepper, celery, snow peas, green beans, and cherry tomatoes. Crunch your way through these goodies or cut larger vegetables into batons and serve alongside hummus or bean dip for added goodness and yum.

Rice or corn cakes make a good substantial snack. Top with nut butters or tahini and sliced banana or fig. Another great option is mashed avocado or edamame beans with sprouts, cherry tomatoes, or leafy greens.

Miso soup is a wonderful pick-me-up that's tasty and so good for you. There are a couple of good instant brands available; be sure to check the ingredients for fish, sometimes labeled as bonito. For a hearty snack, add cubes of tofu or green veggies like asparagus and Brussels sprouts.

SMOOTHIES & JUICES

Including a delicious smoothie or fresh juice in your daily diet is one of the simplest and tastiest ways to pump up your nutrient intake. Great for a midmorning or afternoon snack, they're also perfect for a post-workout fix or a quick-and-nutritious breakfast.

With all the goodness of raw veggies and fruit, just one average glass of fresh juice or smoothie can contain a wealth of vitamins and minerals. Using a high-powered blender, you can whiz up juices as well as smoothies, and the very best blender you can afford will make the job easier. By using a blender you retain all the beneficial fiber from the fruit and vegetables.

Check out the following guides to creating healthy and delicious smoothies—experimenting with different combinations and ingredients is half the fun.

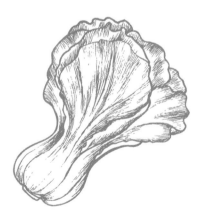

BUILD A FRUIT SMOOTHIE		
	INGREDIENT	AMOUNT
BASE	Apple juice Coconut water	Nondairy milk (almond, rice, oat, or soy)	1–2 cups of any
FRUIT (fresh or frozen)	Avocado Banana Blueberries Cantaloupe Fig Kiwifruit Mango	Nectarine Papaya Peach Pear Raspberries Strawberries	1–2 cups any combination
EXTRAS	Coconut or natural dairy yogurt Ground unsweetened coconut	Nut butter (almond, cashew, peanut, Brazil nut) Rice or seed protein powder	1 tablespoon of any
BOOST IT UP	Cacao powder Chia seeds Flax meal Hemp seeds	Maca powder Probiotic powder Pumpkin seeds Sunflower seeds	1–2 teaspoons any combination
SOMETHING SWEET	Agave syrup Ground cinnamon 1 date, pitted	Honey Maple syrup Pure vanilla extract	½–1 teaspoon of any

Chop up the fruits, throw everything into your blender, and whizz away, adding more base to reach the desired consistency.

Green Smoothies

For a bit more veggie power, try a green smoothie. Adding the nutrient-dense leaves of veggies like spinach and kale to your fruit smoothie really pumps up the goodness. If you work with a ratio of a little more fruit than greens, you won't taste them. It's a great way to add extra green veggies to your diet and perfect for kids too.

BUILD A GREEN SMOOTHIE

	INGREDIENT		AMOUNT
BASE	Coconut water Filtered water	Fresh-squeezed juice (apple, orange, pineapple, watermelon, or cucumber)	1–2 cups of any
FRUIT (fresh or frozen)	Avocado Banana Blueberries Cantaloupe Fig Grapes Kiwi Mango	Nectarine Orange Papaya Peach Pear Raspberries Strawberries	1–2 cups any combination
GREENS	Beet greens Bok choy Kale	Lettuce Parsley Spinach	½–1 cup any combination
BOOST IT UP	Chia seeds Flax meal Ginger, fresh Hemp seeds Mint leaves Probiotic powder	Rice or seed protein powders Spirulina Sunflower seeds Turmeric Wheat grass	1 teaspoon of any
SOMETHING SWEET	Agave syrup Cinnamon, ground 1 date, pitted	Honey Maple syrup Pure vanilla extract	½–1 teaspoon of any

Chop up the fruits, throw everything into your blender, and whiz away, adding more base liquid to reach the desired consistency.

Fresh Fruit & Vegetable Juice

For fresh juices wonderful options are apples, blueberries, raspberries, celery, carrot, orange, lemon, lime, kiwifruit, cantaloupe, watermelon, pineapple, cucumber, beets and beet greens, grapefruit, spinach, kale, fresh ginger, fresh turmeric, mint leaves, parsley, lettuce, and fresh coconut water. Add in spirulina, rice, or seed protein powders and wheat grass for extra goodness. Ice and frozen fruits are great in juices too, making them nice and chilled to serve.

You can make fresh juice in most quality, high-speed blenders; simply add about ½–1 cup of liquid to help get the blender running and easily process the chopped fruit and vegetables. Try filtered water, fresh coconut water, or fresh-squeezed orange juice (you can use a hand juicer to make your own). Avoid hard and fibrous vegetables like carrots and beets, unless you have a juicer or super-high-powered blender, like a Vitamix.

The following are some favorite juice combinations to try:

- Apple, raspberry, beet greens, lime, mint
- Beet, apple, lime, turmeric, mint
- Coconut water, cucumber, pineapple, ginger, parsley
- Orange, carrot, celery, watermelon, ginger

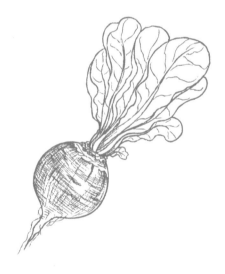

Chapter 4

RECIPES

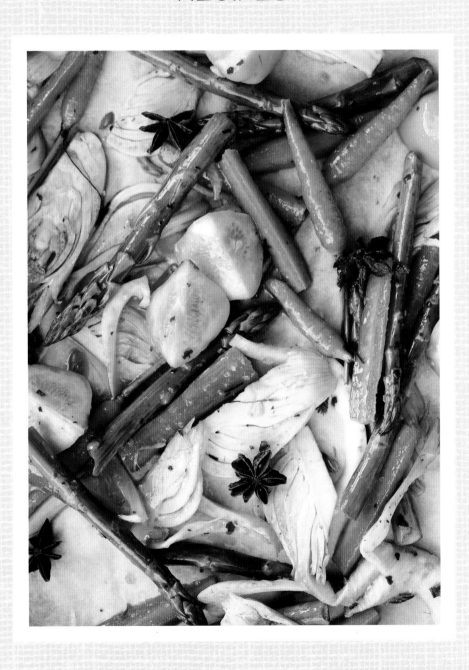

QUICK DRESSINGS & ACCOMPANIMENTS

Sweet Balsamic Dressing

PREP TIME: 2 MINUTES

This is a great all-around dressing, especially good for green leafy salads.

4 tablespoons olive oil

1½ tablespoons balsamic vinegar

½ teaspoon honey or agave nectar

salt flakes and cracked pepper, to taste

Shake ingredients together in a screw top jar until combined.

Szechuan, Sesame Oil, & Lime Dressing

PREP TIME: 2 MINUTES

Serve this dressing over Asian leafy greens; it's particularly good in salads featuring tofu or edamame.

juice from 1 lime

½ tablespoon sesame oil

1½ tablespoons walnut oil

1 teaspoon freshly ground Szechuan peppercorns

pinch of salt flakes

In a screw-top jar combine the dressing ingredients by shaking until smooth.

Caesar(ish) Dressing

PREP TIME: 2 MINUTES

Re-create a Caesar-style salad with this creamy dressing by serving over romaine lettuce and crispy croutons. Also good as a dressing in a cold roast veg salad.

½ cup egg-free or traditional mayonnaise

2 tablespoons olive oil

2 tablespoons fresh apple juice

small squeeze of lemon juice, to taste

¼ teaspoon white miso paste

Whisk all the ingredients together until well combined and smooth.

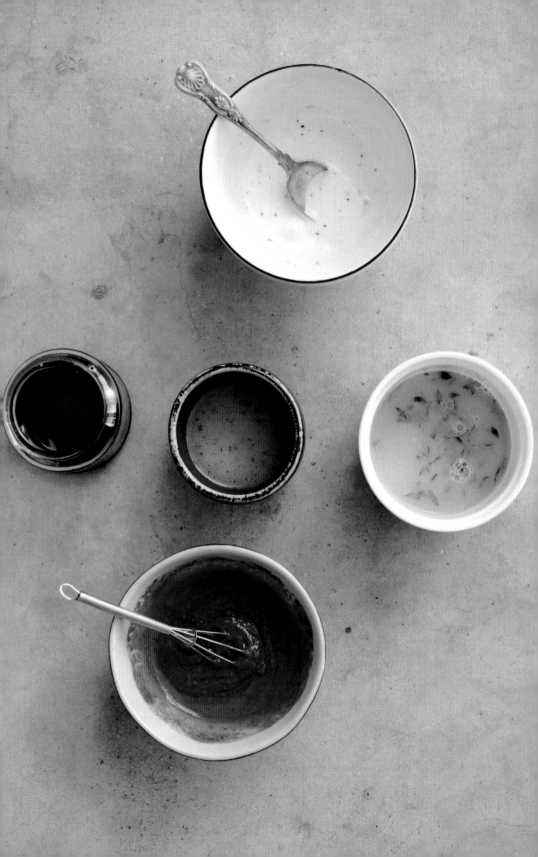

Spicy Almond Dressing

PREP TIME: 2 MINUTES

A spicy dressing that pairs well with roasted vegetables.

1½ tablespoons almond butter

1 tablespoon walnut oil

1 teaspoon balsamic vinegar

½–1 teaspoon harissa

salt flakes and cracked pepper, to taste

Whisk all ingredients together, adding a little water if needed until smooth.

Orange, Honey, and Thyme Dressing

PREP TIME: 2 MINUTES

A lovely light dressing that works well over nearly any
kind of salad; it's particularly good with grains.

zest and juice from 1 orange

2 tablespoons olive oil

1 teaspoon honey (or agave nectar)

1 tablespoon fresh thyme leaves

salt flakes and cracked pepper, to taste

Shake ingredients together in a screw top jar, until combined.

Quick Tomato Relish

PREP TIME: 30 MINUTES • MAKES: ABOUT 2 CUPS

A quick and simple recipe, this tomato relish is perfect for serving in
sandwiches and burgers and with grilled or roasted vegetables.

1 tablespoon sunflower oil

½ tablespoon olive oil

1 red onion, finely diced

2 garlic cloves, minced

1 teaspoon curry powder

1 pound (450 grams) cherry tomatoes (or
any small or medium variety vine-ripened
tomatoes), roughly diced

3 teaspoons brown sugar

2 dried chilies (optional)

¼ cup apple cider vinegar

1. Heat the oils in a heavy frying pan over medium heat. Add the diced onion
   and fry until soft. Add the garlic and curry powder and fry for another minute
   over medium-low heat.

2. Turn up the heat and add the tomatoes, sugar, and dried chilies, if using. Once the tomatoes start to bubble and sizzle, turn down the heat and cook slowly for a few minutes until you can squash the tomatoes with the back of a wooden spoon.

3. Mush the tomatoes to a nice thick pulp, turn up the heat once more, and add the vinegar. Stir together and then cook over low heat for 10–15 minutes until thick and syrupy. Remove from the heat. The relish can be kept covered in the refrigerator for up to a few days.

Kale Pesto

PREP TIME: 5 MINUTES • MAKES: ABOUT 2 CUPS

Try serving this nutritious and tasty pesto in sandwiches and wraps, or spread on rice crackers or toast. It also makes a lovely accompaniment to roasted vegetables.

1 bunch kale, steams removed and roughly chopped

½ cup pine nuts

2 garlic cloves, peeled

¼–½ cup olive oil

salt flakes and cracked pepper

Add the kale, pine nuts, garlic, and the salt flakes and cracked pepper, to taste, to a food processor. With the processor running add the oil a little at a time until you have a rich pesto consistency. Set aside, covered in the refrigerator.

Walnut Paste

PREP TIME: 5 MINUTES + 30 MINUTES REFRIGERATION TIME • MAKES: ABOUT 1 CUP

A delicious accompaniment to grilled or roasted vegetables, it is also nice spread in a wrap or sandwich and topped with leafy greens and sprouts.

1 cup raw walnuts

small bunch fresh thyme

2 teaspoons nutritional yeast

1 dried chili (optional)

juice from ½ lemon

tiny drizzle of honey or agave nectar

2–3 tablespoons walnut or olive oil

salt flakes and cracked pepper

Add all the ingredients except the oil to a food processor, along with salt flakes and cracked pepper, to taste. Process, adding the oil a little at a time until the nuts form a smooth paste. Transfer the walnut paste to a small container and press down until firm. Cover and set aside in the refrigerator.

Tofu-tzatziki

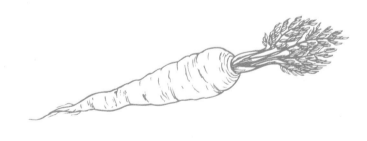

PREP TIME: 10 MINUTES • SERVES: 4

Serve this with raw vegetables for dipping, on wraps, in
sandwiches, or with a Middle Eastern platter.

KID-APPROVED • SOY PROTEIN • DIFFICULTY LEVEL*

1 Persian cucumber

1 tablespoon olive oil

1 garlic clove, minced

¼ teaspoon dill seeds (optional)

zest and juice from 1 lemon

10 ounces (300 grams) silken tofu

salt flakes and cracked pepper

1. Peel and finely grate the cucumber. Squeeze the grated cucumber in your hand
   to remove the excess liquid. Place in a small bowl and set aside.

2. Heat the oil over a medium-low heat in a small pan. Add the garlic and dill
   seeds and fry gently for 1–2 minutes until fragrant. Add the lemon zest and
   fry for another 30 seconds and then remove from the heat and cool.

3. Place the silken tofu into a food processor; add the olive oil, garlic, dill, and
   lemon zest from the pan. Squeeze about half the lemon juice over the mixture
   and process until smooth. Taste, adding salt flakes, cracked pepper and more
   lemon juice as needed. Transfer to the bowl with the grated cucumber and
   fold through.

4. Keeps well-covered in the refrigerator for a day or two.

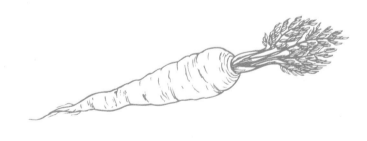

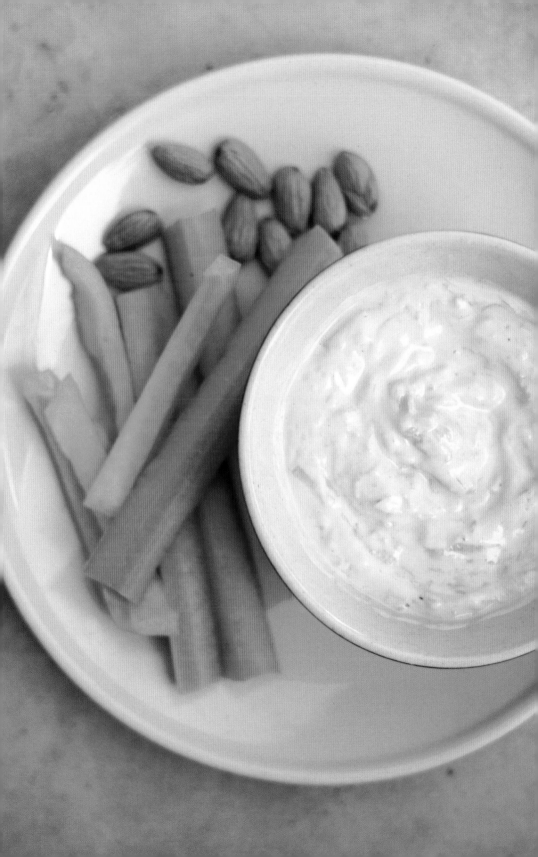

BREAKFASTS & SWEET TREATS

Coco Banana Overnight Oats

PREP TIME: 5 MINUTES + OVERNIGHT TO SOAK • SERVES: 1

Try any combination of fresh, stewed, or dried fruits, nuts, and seeds you can think of. You can even use honey or fruit juice in place of the maple syrup. If you plan to take the oats in the morning to eat on the go, simply prepare them in a sealed container or glass jar and top with any granola or fresh fruits before you head out.

KID-APPROVED • DIFFICULTY LEVEL *

⅓ cup rolled oats

⅓ cup rice, soy, or almond milk

⅓ cup coconut yogurt (or natural dairy yogurt)

1 teaspoon chia seeds

1 teaspoon maple syrup

¼ teaspoon pure vanilla extract (optional)

½ banana, sliced

fresh fruit, crunchy toasted granola, nut butter, or seeds, for garnish

Combine the first seven ingredients together in a bowl, cover, and place in the fridge overnight. Serve in the morning as is or topped with fresh fruit, some crunchy toasted granola, nut butter, or seeds.

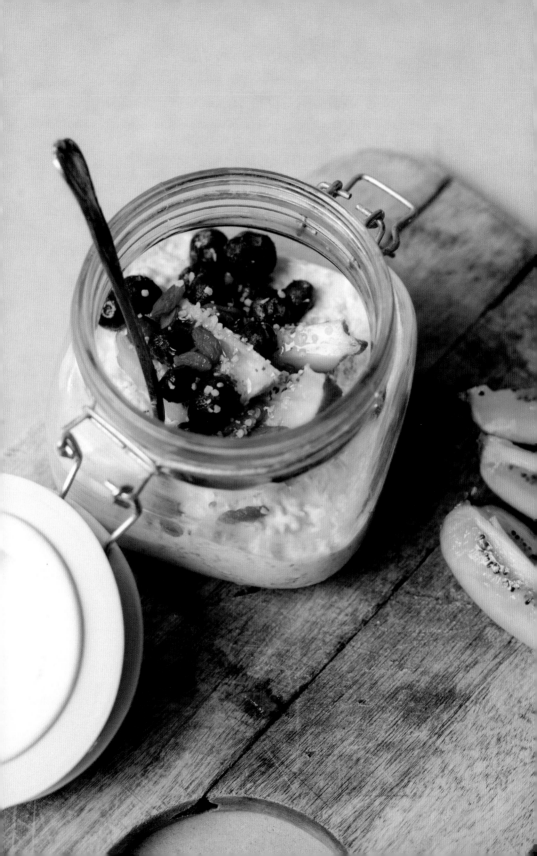

Breakfast Smoothie

PREP TIME: 5 MINUTES • SERVES: 1–2

Fruit smoothies are really only limited by your imagination. Add any combination of fresh or frozen fruits to make your own version. Try experimenting with fresh, pitted dates for sweetness and rice or seed protein powders, flax, sunflower or pumpkin seeds, and ground coconut for added nutrition and yum. Frozen bananas are fantastic in smoothies, adding a delectable creaminess. Simply throw whole ripe bananas in the freezer for use later on. To use, run them under the tap for a few seconds before sliding a knife down the skins to peel.

KID-APPROVED • PERFECT FOR NEW VEGETARIANS • DIFFICULTY LEVEL *

1 cup rice, soy, or almond milk

1 fig or kiwifruit, quartered, or a small handful of fresh or frozen berries

1 fresh or frozen banana

1 tablespoon almond butter or tahini

1 teaspoon cacao powder

1 teaspoon chia seeds

¼ teaspoon ground cinnamon

Blend all ingredients together in a high-powered blender. Serve immediately.

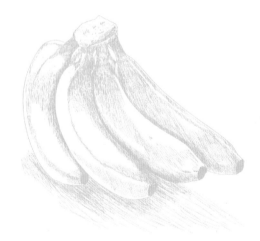

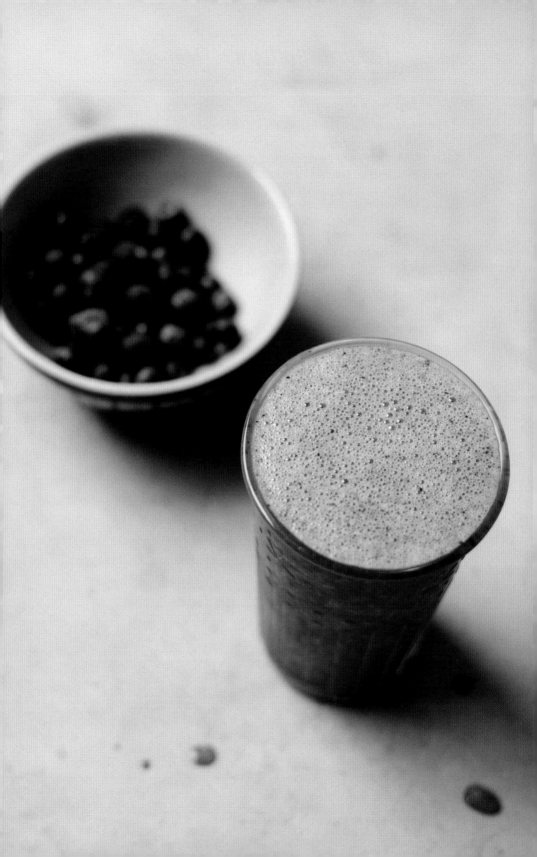

Toasted Multigrain Granola

PREP TIME: 25 MINUTES • SERVES: 12 (MAKES ABOUT 6 CUPS)

Use this recipe as a guide to making your own toasted or natural granola with your favorite ingredients, swapping out the oats for things like quinoa flakes or rolled spelt and the buckwheat groats for puffed amaranth or puffed rice. Try any combination of seeds, nuts, and dried fruits of your choice.

WHOLE-GRAIN GOODNESS • PERFECT FOR NEW
VEGETARIANS • DIFFICULTY LEVEL **

1 cup raw buckwheat groats

1 cup rolled oats

1 cup rolled rye

1 cup dried apricots or figs (look for sulphate/preservative free)

½ cup shredded coconut

½ cup sunflower seeds

½ cup pumpkin seeds

¼ cup flaxseeds (linseeds)

2 teaspoons ground cinnamon

¼ cup maple syrup

3 tablespoons virgin (cold-pressed) coconut oil

1. Preheat the oven to 300°F (150°C) and line two large baking trays with baking paper.

2. Mix all the dry ingredients together in a large bowl, tossing to combine well. Pour the maple syrup and coconut oil over the mixture and toss again until everything is coated with the oil and syrup.

3. Pour the mixture in an even layer over both the baking trays. Pop in the oven and toast for 15 minutes until golden.

4. Remove from the oven and allow to cool completely on the trays before transferring to a sealed jar or container. The toasted granola should keep well for up to two weeks in your pantry.

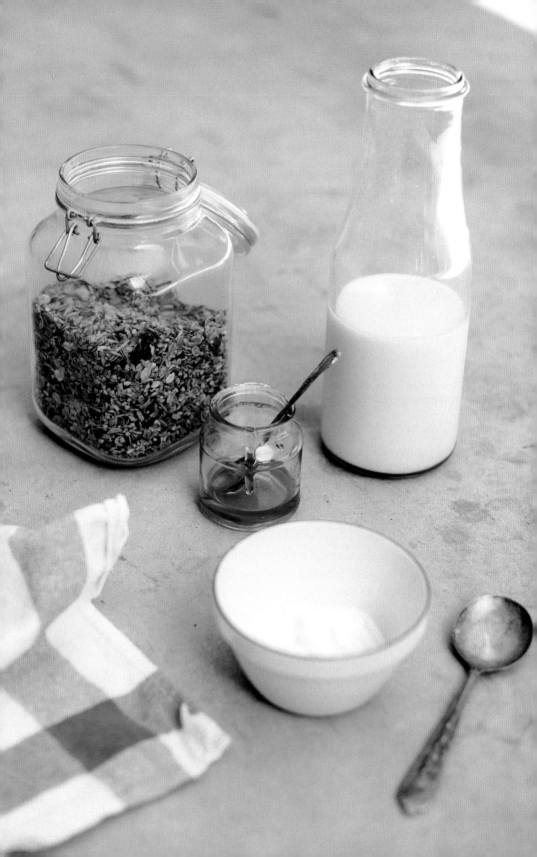

Whole Wheat/Spelt Pancakes

PREP TIME: 30 MINUTES • SERVES: 2–4

Try adding 1 tablespoon of cacao powder, flax meal, or ground coconut on top of the sifted flours for added nutrition. Serve topped with seasonal fresh fruits, shredded coconut, seeds, nut butters, and/or a drizzle of maple or coconut syrup. For a non-vegan version, swap the coconut butter for melted dairy butter and the chia gel for one certified free-range egg.

> WHOLE-GRAIN GOODNESS • KID-APPROVED • PERFECT
> FOR NEW VEGETARIANS • DIFFICULTY LEVEL **

1 teaspoon chia seeds

¼ cup water

1 cup spelt flour

¼ cup self-rising whole wheat flour

1½ teaspoons baking powder

¼ cup virgin (cold-pressed) coconut oil

1 tablespoon maple syrup

½ teaspoon vanilla bean paste

1¼ cups rice, soy, or oat milk

1. In a small bowl combine the chia seeds with the water and set aside for at least 10 minutes until it forms a runny, jelly-like consistency similar to raw egg.

2. Sift the flours and baking powder into a large bowl.

3. Soften the coconut oil until translucent and runny (either by warming in a small saucepan over low heat or carefully microwaving, in a small glass or ceramic bowl, on low for 10 seconds).

4. In a small bowl combine the softened coconut oil with the maple syrup and vanilla bean paste.

5. Make a well in the center of the flour mixture. Gradually add the cooled coconut oil mixture, followed by the milk and the chia gel, whisking to form a smooth batter. Add more milk if you prefer a runnier batter.

6. In a large heavy pan, heat a small amount of neutral oil, like sunflower, over medium heat.

7. Add spoonfuls of the batter to the pan. Watch for bubbles to appear on the top surface of the pancakes before flipping them over to cook the other side. Keep cooked pancakes warm in a low oven while you prepare the remainder.

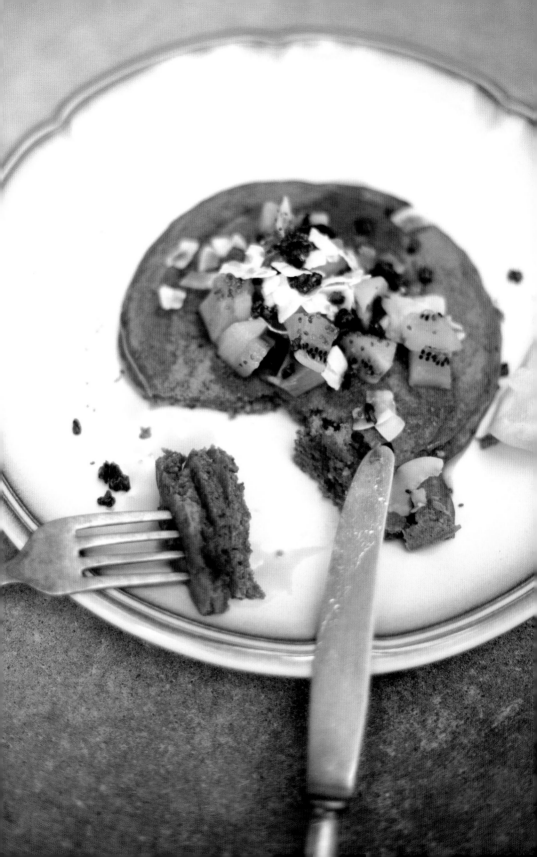

Seeded Banana Bread with Dried Figs and Turkish Apricots

PREP TIME: 55 MINUTES • MAKES: 1 LOAF

Try making this banana bread with your favorite seeds and dried fruits or use a combination of nuts and seeds. Walnuts, flaked almonds, pistachios, hazelnuts, and pecans would all be good.

KID-APPROVED • WHOLE-GRAIN GOODNESS • DIFFICULTY LEVEL *

2 teaspoons chia seeds

½ cup water

1 cup plain unbleached flour

¼ cup spelt or amaranth flour

3 teaspoons baking powder

1 teaspoon ground cinnamon

1 teaspoon ground cardamom

¼ cup flaxseeds (linseeds)

¼ cup sunflower seeds

¼ cup raw sugar

1 ½ cups (about 2–3) mashed over-ripe banana

¼ cup sunflower oil

1 teaspoon pure vanilla extract

¼ cup dried figs, roughly diced

¼ cup Turkish apricots, roughly diced

1 teaspoon pumpkin seeds

1. In a small bowl combine the chia seeds with the water and set aside for at least 10 minutes until it forms a runny, jelly-like consistency similar to raw egg.

2. Preheat the oven to 350°F (180°C) and grease and line an 8 x 4½-inch (20 x 11-centimeter) loaf pan.

3. Sift the flours and baking powder into a large bowl. Add the spices, seeds (except the pumpkin seeds), and sugar, and stir to combine.

4. In a small bowl combine the mashed banana with the oil, chia gel, and vanilla. Whisk until smooth.

5. Add the wet ingredients to the dry and stir until just combined. Add the dried fruits and fold through.

6. Pour the mixture into the prepared loaf pan and scatter the pumpkin seeds on top.

7. Place in the preheated oven and bake for 40 minutes until lightly golden and cooked through (check with a skewer inserted into the middle of the bread). Remove from the oven and cool for 5 minutes in the pan before transferring to a wire rack to cool completely.

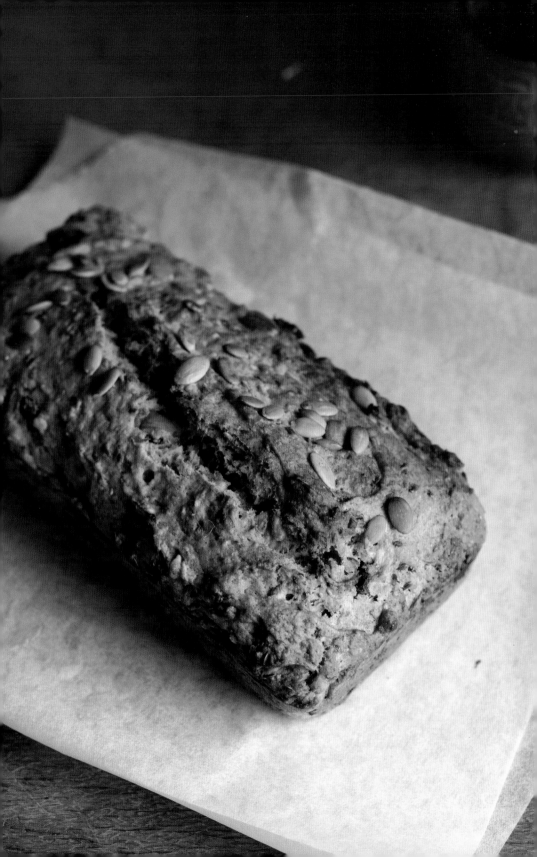

Whole-Grain Cacao Chip Cookies

PREP TIME: 15 MINUTES • MAKES: ABOUT 20 COOKIES

You can substitute any nut butter you prefer in place of the peanut butter. They are particularly good with ABC (almond, Brazil nut, and cashew) butter. Experiment by replacing the amaranth flour with different whole-grain flours, too—try whole wheat, oat, or even buckwheat.

KID-APPROVED • WHOLE-GRAIN GOODNESS • DIFFICULTY LEVEL *

½ cup self-rising whole wheat flour

½ cup amaranth flour

1 ½ cup quinoa flakes

¼ cup almond meal

½ cup brown sugar

¼ cup cacao nibs

3½ ounces (100 grams) smooth raw peanut butter (or nut butter of your choice)

¼ cup hot water

2 tablespoons maple syrup

½ teaspoon baking soda

2 tablespoons warm water

1. Preheat the oven to 350°F (180°C).

2. Line two baking trays with baking paper and set aside.

3. Combine the dry ingredients well in a large bowl, using your fingers if necessary to break up the brown sugar.

4. In a small bowl add the peanut butter, maple syrup, and about half the hot water. Whisk the peanut butter and syrup with the water, adding more water when necessary until the mixture is smooth and resembles a thick syrup; you may need more or less than the ¼ cup of water, so add it gradually.

5. In a small bowl mix the baking soda with the 2 tablespoons of warm water until it has dissolved; add to the peanut butter mixture and stir through.

6. Add the peanut butter and maple syrup mixture to the dry ingredients and combine well. The cookie dough should be soft, moist, and a little sticky; you can add a little extra maple syrup if you feel it is too dry.

7. Roll about 1 small tablespoon of the mixture into a ball and place on the prepared baking tray. Lightly press each cookie down carefully with the back of a fork.

8. Place in the preheated oven and bake for 8–12 minutes; watch them carefully and remove from the oven just as they start to turn very lightly golden.

9. Allow them to rest on the baking tray for 5 minutes before placing on a wire rack to cool.

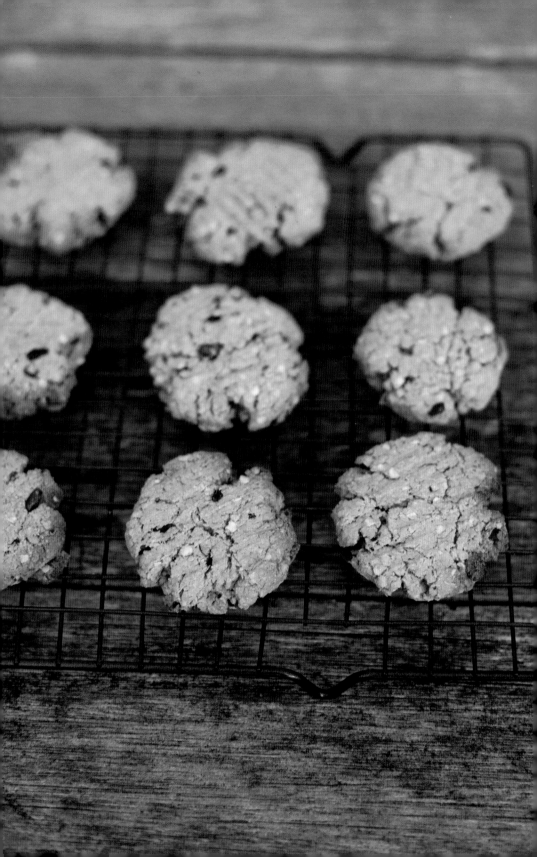

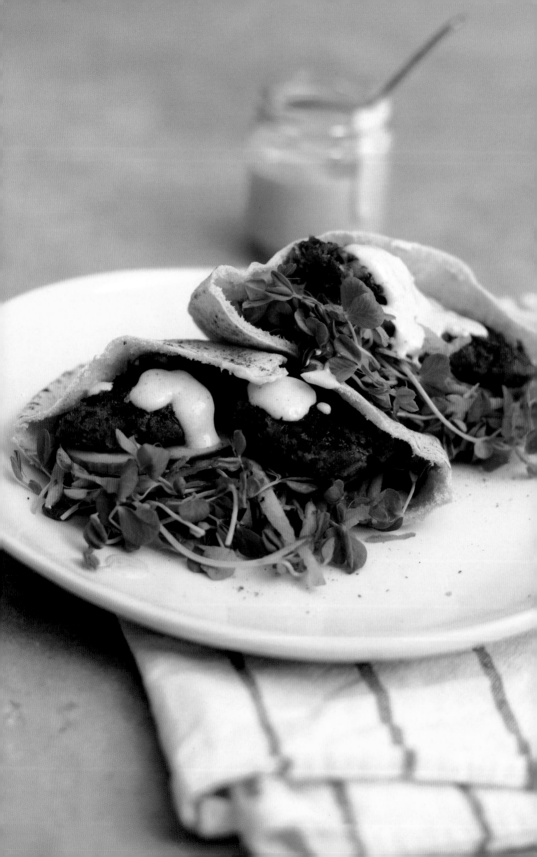

LIGHTER MEALS

Pita Pockets with Carrot Falafel and Creamy Harissa Sauce

PREP TIME: 45 MINUTES • SERVES: 4

If you prefer a milder sauce, use tomato paste instead of harissa. The falafel also make a great burger—try serving in toasted Turkish bread or seeded buns instead of the pita bread. This recipe should make about eight good-sized falafel or small patties. If serving to a larger group, simply double the recipe.

> PERFECT FOR NEW VEGETARIANS • KID-APPROVED •
> PACKED WITH VEGGIE POWER • LEGUME PROTEIN •
> GREAT FOR ENTERTAINING • DIFFICULTY LEVEL **

CARROT FALAFELS

1½ cups (about 2 large) carrots, sliced into thick rounds

½ red onion, peeled and cut into two wedges

1 tablespoon olive oil

1 teaspoon cumin seeds

½ teaspoon smoked paprika

½ teaspoon high-quality curry powder

1½ tablespoons rolled rye or oats

1 tablespoon sunflower seeds

1 cup cilantro, roughly chopped

1 cup flat-leaf parsley, roughly chopped

1½ cups cooked or canned chickpeas, rinsed well

½ cup golden raisins

salt flakes and cracked pepper

CREAMY HARISSA SAUCE

¾ cup silken tofu

juice from 1 lemon

1 tablespoon olive oil

1–2 teaspoons harissa, to taste

¼ teaspoon maple syrup

ADDITIONAL INGREDIENTS

1–2 tablespoons sunflower oil for frying

4 whole wheat pita breads, warmed in a low oven

snow pea sprouts (plus extra for garnish), sliced cucumber, or grated carrot

1. Preheat the oven to 400°F (200°C).

2. Arrange the chopped carrot and wedges of onion on a baking tray. Drizzle with the olive oil, sprinkle the spices on top, along with salt flakes and cracked pepper, to taste, and then toss to coat well.

3. Place in the preheated oven for 25–30 minutes, until the carrot is golden and tender. Remove from the oven and allow to cool.

4. Meanwhile, in a food processor, process the rolled rye or oats and sunflower seeds to form a coarse flour. Add the fresh herbs and process for a few seconds until finely chopped.

5. Add the chickpeas, golden raisins, roasted carrot, and onions, along with all the oil and spices in the bottom of the roasting pan, to the flour mixture in the food processor.

6. Using the pulse setting, pulse the ingredients until they just start to come together. Be sure not to overprocess the ingredients—you want to keep some texture and not end up with a mixture that resembles hummus.

7. Using clean hands, form a large tablespoon of falafel mixture into a ball and then flatten slightly into a small round patty. Repeat with the remaining mixture (the falafels can be made ahead of time and stored, covered in the refrigerator).

8. Prepare the creamy harissa sauce by blending all the ingredients together, either using a stick blender or a small food processor, until smooth. Set aside.

9. To fry the falafel, heat a small amount of sunflower oil in a heavy frying or grill pan. Alternatively, you can cook the patties on a barbecue grill. Working in small batches, fry the falafels over medium-high heat, turning once golden on one side to cook on the other. Remove from the pan, place on paper towels, and keep warm while you cook the remainder.

10. Serve the falafel immediately, piled into the warm pita pockets with lots of sprouts, cucumber, grated carrot, and a good drizzle of the creamy harissa sauce.

Grilled Mushrooms on Rye with Fresh Tomato Salsa and Creamy Horseradish Sauce

PREP TIME: 35 MINUTES • SERVES: 4

If using fresh horseradish, reduce the amount, adding a little at a time. Alternatively, try whole-grain mustard. Use arugula or cress in place of the sprouts if you prefer. This recipe also makes a great veggie burger with a seeded bun instead of the rye.

PERFECT FOR NEW VEGETARIANS • PACKED WITH VEGGIE POWER • GREAT FOR ENTERTAINING • DIFFICULTY LEVEL *

GRILLED GARLIC MUSHROOMS

1 pound (450 grams) portobello mushrooms

3 tablespoons olive oil

3 garlic cloves, minced

1–2 teaspoons chili flakes (optional)

2 teaspoons fresh thyme leaves

1 tablespoon sunflower oil

salt flakes and cracked pepper

FRESH CHERRY TOMATO SALSA

7 ounces (200 grams) cherry tomatoes, sliced

½ green bell pepper, finely diced

2 teaspoons finely diced red onion

1–2 tablespoons torn fresh basil leaves

pinch of raw sugar

salt flakes and cracked pepper, to taste

CREAMY HORSERADISH SAUCE

¾ cup silken tofu

2 tablespoons lemon juice

½ teaspoon brown sugar

1 tablespoon walnut oil or olive oil

1–3 teaspoons fresh horseradish or horseradish cream to taste

salt flakes and cracked pepper, to taste

ADDITIONAL INGREDIENTS

8 slices of dark rye bread, toasted

good bunch of fresh snow pea or alfalfa sprouts

1. Slice the mushrooms into thick (approximately ⅓-inch/1 cm) slices.

2. Place the mushroom slices in a single layer in a large shallow container, drizzle the olive oil on top, along with the crushed garlic, chili flakes, and fresh thyme. Season with salt flakes and fresh cracked pepper, to taste, and then toss to coat evenly. Cover and set aside in the refrigerator while you prepare the remainder of the ingredients.

3. To make the salsa, combine all the ingredients together in a small bowl and toss well, adding salt flakes and cracked pepper to taste. Set aside in the refrigerator.

4. For the creamy horseradish sauce, place the silken tofu, lemon juice, and brown sugar in a food processor. With the motor running, add the oil until the tofu becomes a smooth cream. Add a little of the horseradish at a time, adjusting to taste, and finish with a little pinch of salt flakes and cracked pepper. Set aside in the refrigerator.

5. To cook the mushrooms, heat a small amount of the sunflower oil on a grill, griddle, or heavy frying pan. Grill the mushrooms in small batches over a medium-high heat until golden on both sides. Set aside and keep warm while you cook the remainder.

6. Assemble the sandwich by spreading all slices of toasted rye with the horseradish sauce. Top each of the four slices with sprouts, a nice stack of grilled mushrooms, and spoonfuls of salsa, and finish with the second slice of rye.

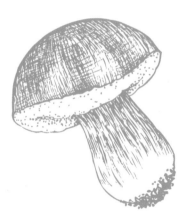

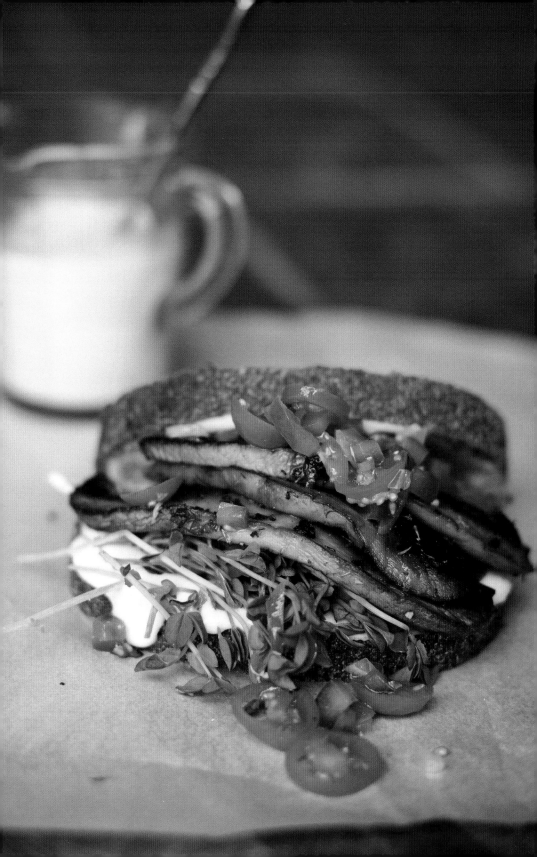

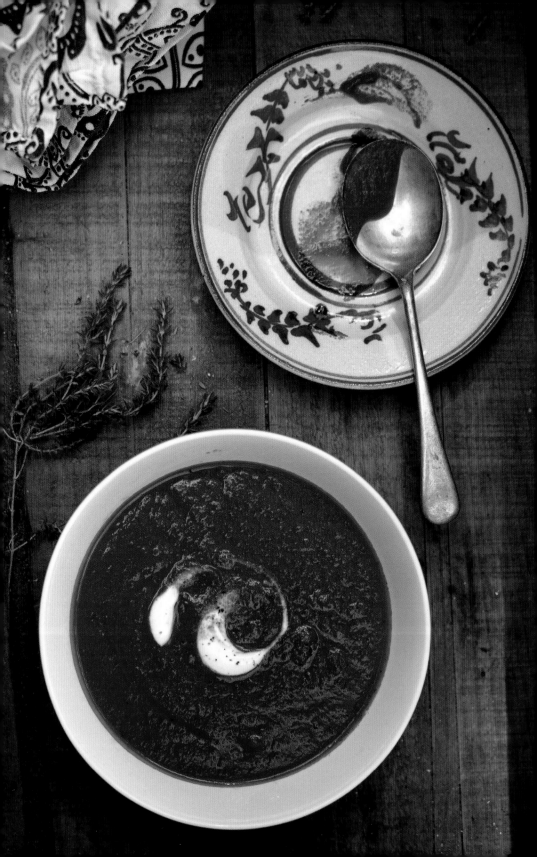

Super Beet Soup with Apple, Celery, and Turmeric

PREP TIME: 50 MINUTES • SERVES: 4

If you can't find fresh turmeric root, substitute with around 2 teaspoons of ground turmeric, adding it along with the ground cumin and cinnamon. Fresh ginger is also lovely as a substitute to the fresh turmeric.

KID-APPROVED • PACKED WITH VEGGIE POWER • DIFFICULTY LEVEL *

2 tablespoons sunflower oil

4 pearl onions, peeled and diced

3 celery stalks and leafy tops, chopped

1 teaspoon ground cumin

¼ teaspoon ground cinnamon

2 large beets, scrubbed and cubed

2 red skinned apples, cored and cubed

1 good teaspoon grated fresh turmeric root

4 cups vegetable stock

2 cups water

ADDITIONAL INGREDIENTS

lemon wedges

soy or natural plain yogurt

dark rye bread

1. Heat the oil over medium heat in a large deep saucepan.

2. Add the diced onions and chopped celery stalks (reserving the leafy tops) and cook for a few minutes until the onion is soft.

3. Add the ground cumin and cinnamon and toss through over medium heat until fragrant and dissolved. Be careful not to have the heat too high, as this may burn the spices.

4. Add the diced beets, apples, and grated fresh turmeric. Toss through for a few minutes and then turn up the heat.

5. Add the celery tops, stock, and water and bring to a simmer.

6. Turn down the heat and gently simmer for around 35 minutes until the beets are tender. Remove from the heat.

7. Using a stick blender, or carefully in batches in a food processor, blend the soup until smooth. Return to the heat and warm through.

8. Serve with a squeeze of lemon juice, a swirl of soy or natural yogurt, and a side of crusty bread for dunking.

Satay Tempeh Lettuce Wraps

PREP TIME: 45 MINUTES • MAKES: ABOUT 8 LETTUCE WRAPS

The pickles are best made the day before and will keep in the refrigerator for a few days. You can prepare the satay skewers ahead of time and keep covered overnight in the refrigerator. This recipe is also great served in bread rolls as a vegetarian bahn mi.

PERFECT FOR NEW VEGETARIANS • PACKED WITH VEGGIE POWER • SOY PROTEIN • GREAT FOR ENTERTAINING • DIFFICULTY LEVEL **

PICKLED CARROT, CUCUMBER, AND CHILI

½ cup rice wine vinegar

¼–½ teaspoon brown sugar, to taste

1 carrot, thinly sliced

1 Persian cucumber, thinly sliced

1 green chili, thinly sliced (optional)

SATAY TEMPEH SKEWERS

1 tablespoon peanut oil

2 garlic cloves, minced

1 chili, diced (optional)

1 teaspoon curry powder or paste

2 tablespoons raw peanut butter

2 teaspoons palm sugar

1 cup light coconut milk

1 lime

1 pound (450 grams) tempeh

ADDITIONAL INGREDIENTS

sunflower oil, for grilling

2 heads romaine or iceberg lettuce, leaves separated

3 cups bean sprouts, washed

½ cup roughly chopped cilantro

egg-free mayonnaise, to serve

1. Make the pickles by heating the vinegar in a small saucepan over medium-low heat until warm. Remove from the heat and stir the brown sugar in until dissolved. Place the sliced vegetables in a jar, pouring the vinegar mixture over them.

2. Set aside in the refrigerator, shaking the jar every now and then.

3. For the satay sauce, heat the peanut oil over a medium heat in a heavy frying pan. Add the garlic and chili, if using, and fry for 1 minute; add the curry powder and stir to combine with the oil.

4. Add the peanut butter, palm sugar, and coconut milk. Turn down the heat and cook at a low simmer for a few minutes, stirring until smooth. Add a good squeeze of lime juice and remove from the heat.

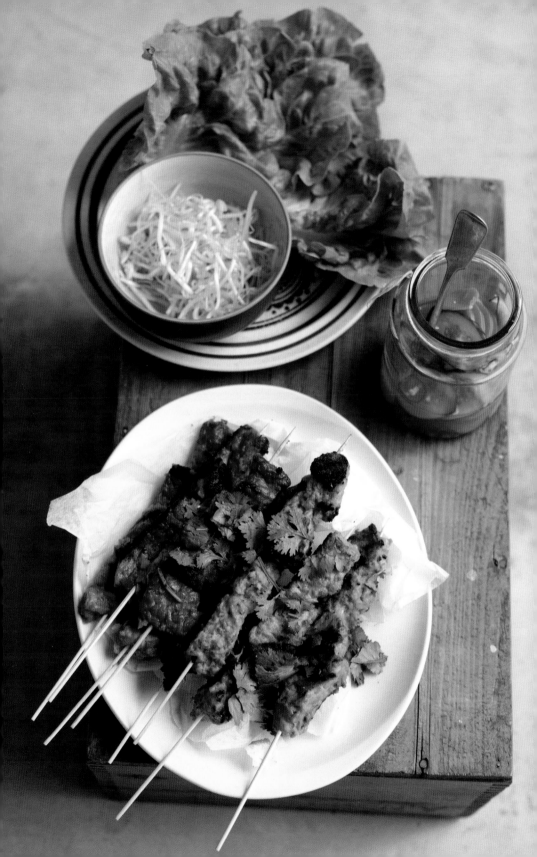

5. Tear the tempeh into bite-size chunks and toss in the prepared satay sauce until well coated. Thread the tempeh pieces onto each of eight bamboo or metal skewers. Reserve any remaining satay sauce for serving.

6. To grill the tempeh skewers, heat a small amount of oil on a barbecue grill or stovetop grill pan. Grill the prepared tempeh skewers over medium-high heat, turning until golden on all sides. Keep warm.

7. To serve, remove the tempeh from the skewers and slice into smaller pieces if you prefer. Allow everyone to fill their own lettuce wraps with the torn cilantro, bean sprouts, pickles, and tempeh, adding a little mayonnaise and reserved satay sauce drizzled over the top.

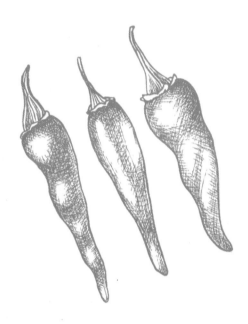

Soba Noodles and Sesame-Ginger Greens with Shiitake-Miso Broth

PREP TIME: 25 MINUTES • SERVES: 4

Use your favorite in-season vegetables here—Brussels sprouts, snow peas, beans, edamame, broccoli, and any of the Asian greens would all be lovely. If you can't find fresh shiitake mushrooms, substitute with what's available, or try bamboo shoots or lotus root instead.

PACKED WITH VEGGIE POWER • WHOLE-GRAIN
GOODNESS • DIFFICULTY LEVEL *

SHIITAKE-MISO BROTH

6 whole dried shiitake mushrooms

1 cup vegetable stock

1 ½ cups water

2 teaspoons miso paste

SESAME-GINGER GREENS

2 baby bok choy

1 bunch asparagus

3½ ounces (100 grams) fresh shiitake mushrooms

1 tablespoon sesame oil

1 tablespoon sunflower oil

2-inch (5-centimeter) piece of fresh ginger, finely grated

2 garlic cloves, minced

1 tablespoon sesame seeds

½–1 teaspoon chili flakes (optional)

1 teaspoon tamari or soy sauce, or to taste

ADDITIONAL INGREDIENTS

3½ ounces (100 grams) soba noodles

1. Prepare the miso broth by adding all the ingredients to a small saucepan. Bring to a gentle simmer and cook over medium-low heat, simmering for 10 minutes. Before serving, remove the whole mushrooms and reserve for later.

2. Meanwhile bring water to boil in a medium saucepan. Once boiling, add the soba noodles and cook rapidly for 4 minutes. Strain and rinse with cold water briefly. Set aside.

3. Chop the ends from the baby bok choy, snap the woody ends off the asparagus, and roughly slice the shiitake mushrooms used for the broth.

4. To stir-fry the vegetables, heat the sesame and sunflower oils in a heavy frying pan or wok over medium-high heat. Add the ginger, garlic, sesame seeds, and chili, if using. Fry for just a minute until fragrant, then add the mushrooms, tossing for a few minutes before adding the bok choy and asparagus, seasoning with soy sauce to taste.

5. Toss quickly, until combined and the bok choy is just wilted. Remove from the heat and serve immediately accompanied by the hot miso broth and noodles.

6. To serve, divide the noodles among four bowls, top with the stir-fried vegetables, and then pour a little hot broth on top.

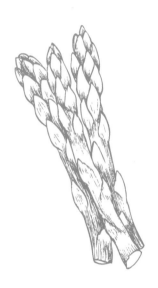

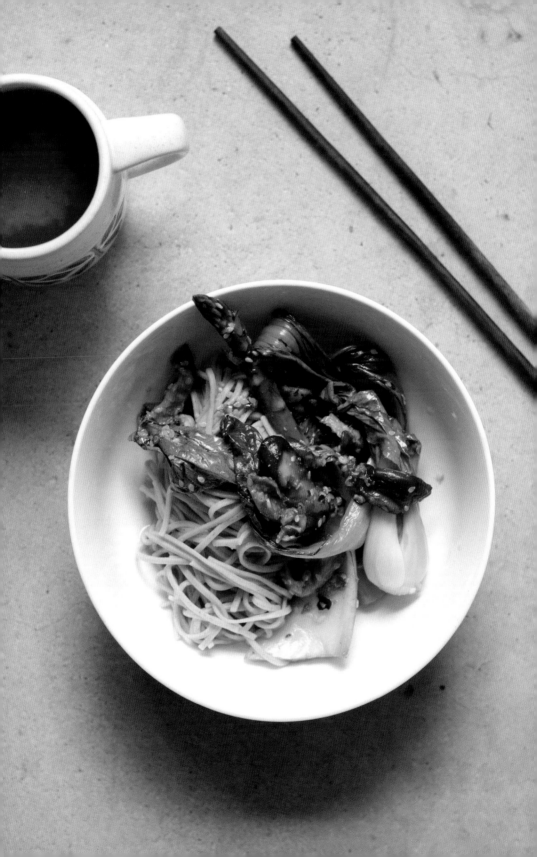

Warm Vegetable and Barley Salad with Orange, Honey, and Thyme Dressing

PREP TIME: 45 MINUTES • SERVES: 4–6

If you enjoy dairy, try serving strips of grilled vegetarian halloumi on top.
Cube the pumpkin slightly larger than the sweet potato as it cooks faster.

PERFECT FOR NEW VEGETARIANS • PACKED WITH VEGGIE
POWER • WHOLE-GRAIN GOODNESS • DIFFICULTY LEVEL *

SALAD

¾ cup pearl barley

1-pound (450-gram) piece of pumpkin, cubed

1-pound (450-gram) piece of sweet potato, scrubbed and cubed

3 tablespoons olive oil

1 tablespoon raw honey, agave nectar, or maple syrup

1 teaspoon cumin seeds

1 teaspoon black cumin seeds (optional)

¼ cup pumpkin seeds

2 cups baby spinach

2 cups arugula

DRESSING

zest and juice from 1 orange

2 tablespoons olive oil

1 teaspoon honey or agave nectar

1 tablespoon chopped fresh thyme

salt flakes and cracked pepper, to taste

1. Preheat the oven to 400°F (200°C).

2. Rinse the barley well and place in a good-sized pot with 3 cups of water. Gently boil, covered, for approximately 35 minutes until all the water is absorbed and the barley is tender. Keep warm.

3. Place the cubed pumpkin and sweet potato on a baking tray. Drizzle with the olive oil and honey, agave, or maple syrup, scattering the cumin on top. Toss to coat well and then roast in the preheated oven for 30–35 minutes until golden. Keep warm.

4. Meanwhile dry roast the pumpkin seeds in a small frying pan over a medium-low heat. Watch them carefully and toss frequently. In just a minute or two they'll start to turn golden and pop. Remove from the heat.

5. Prepare the dressing by whisking all the ingredients together with salt flakes and freshly cracked pepper until combined.

6. To prepare the salad, toss the cooked barley with the vegetables, spinach, arugula, and roasted pumpkin seeds, and toss the dressing through just before serving.

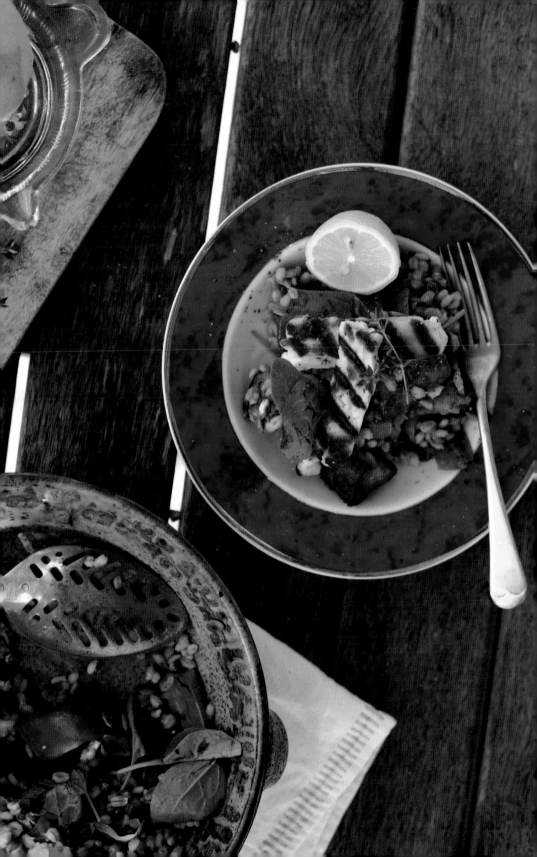

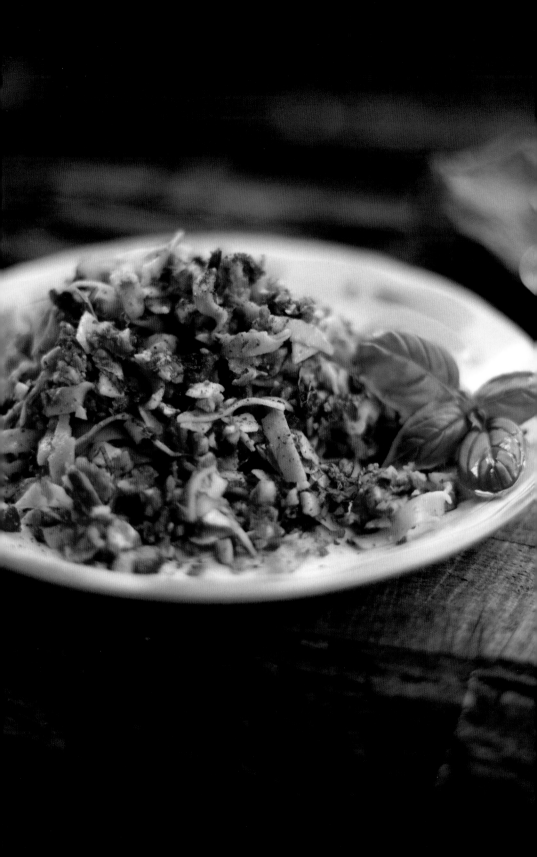

WHOLESOME DINNERS

Roasted Eggplant and Almond Pesto with Whole Wheat Pasta

PREP TIME: 75 MINUTES • SERVES: 4

This beautiful pesto is full of robust flavor and makes a great topping for bruschetta as well as served with pasta. Make ahead and store covered in the refrigerator for a quick midweek meal. Strict vegetarians should omit the vegetarian feta cheese and choose one of the many egg-free pasta varieties available.

PACKED WITH VEGGIE POWER • WHOLE-GRAIN GOODNESS • GREAT FOR ENTERTAINING • DIFFICULTY LEVEL **

ROASTED EGGPLANT AND ALMOND PESTO WITH SUNDRIED TOMATOES AND SUMAC

2 pounds (1 kilogram) eggplant (approximately 2 large eggplants)

salt flakes

2 tablespoons olive oil

7 ounces (200 grams) raw almonds

7-ounce (200-gram) jar of quality sundried tomatoes in olive oil

½ cup golden raisins

1 good handful of fresh herbs (mint, basil, and parsley)

2 teaspoons sumac

cracked pepper

ADDITIONAL INGREDIENTS

9 ounces (250 grams) whole wheat fettuccine or tagliatelle (or an egg-free alternative)

salt, for pasta water

2–3 tablespoons olive oil, divided

2 garlic cloves, minced

zest and juice from 1 lemon

1 cup of vegetarian feta cheese (optional)

1. Preheat the oven to 350°F (180°C).

2. Slice the eggplant lengthways into approximately ½-inch (1.5-centimeter) rounds.

3. Lay the slices in a colander, sprinkling lightly with salt flakes between the layers. Once the eggplant slices begin to sweat, around 10–20 minutes, remove from the colander and pat dry on a clean tea towel or paper towel.

4. Brush two large baking trays with olive oil. Arrange the slices of eggplant on the trays and brush with more olive oil. Roast in the preheated oven for 30–35 minutes until soft and golden. Remove and allow to cool.

5. Meanwhile, dry roast the almonds over low heat in a pan. Remove and set aside to cool.

6. Using a food processor, blend the sundried tomatoes with their oil and the raisins to a coarse paste. Transfer to a large bowl.

7. Using the same food processor, blend the almonds coarsely with the fresh herbs and then add to the sundried tomato mixture.

8. Add the cooled roasted eggplant to the food processor and blend to a thick, chunky pulp. Transfer to the bowl with the processed almonds, herbs, and sundried tomatoes.

9. Add the sumac, season with salt flakes and cracked pepper, to taste, and stir to combine well. Set aside. Pesto can be made ahead of time and stored covered in the refrigerator for up to 2 days.

10. To make the pasta, bring a large pot of lightly salted water to a boil. Cook the pasta in rapidly boiling water according to the packet instructions.

11. Meanwhile heat 1 tablespoon of the olive oil in a large frying pan. Add the garlic and fry over a medium-low heat for a minute until fragrant. Add the cooked and drained pasta, tossing with the garlic and oil before adding the prepared pesto.

12. Toss the pasta and pesto over medium-low heat to coat evenly and until thoroughly heated through.

13. Remove from the heat and toss through the lemon zest and a little lemon juice to taste. Before serving, drizzle with a little extra olive oil and toss the feta through, if using.

14. Serve sprinkled with a little extra sumac, if desired.

Mushroom Cannelloni with Cauliflower Béchamel

PREP TIME: 1 HOUR, 10 MINUTES • SERVES: 6

For a really gooey, cheesy sauce, add nondairy or dairy cheese
to the cauliflower béchamel. A little vegetarian Parmesan-style
cheese is nice grated over the top to get that lovely golden-brown
color; or substitute with a nondairy cheese of your choice.

PERFECT FOR NEW VEGETARIANS • PACKED WITH VEGGIE POWER
• GREAT FOR ENTERTAINING • DIFFICULTY LEVEL ***

CAULIFLOWER BÉCHAMEL

2 tablespoons sunflower oil

1 large head of cauliflower, thinly sliced

½ teaspoon paprika

salt flakes, to taste

¾ cup nondairy milk of your choice

¼ teaspoon ground nutmeg

3 teaspoons nutritional yeast (optional)

cracked pepper

juice from 1 lemon, to taste

1–2 cups nondairy or dairy cheese (optional)

MUSHROOM CANNELLONI

7 ounces (200 grams) button mushrooms

7 ounces (200 grams) brown mushrooms

3½ ounces (100 grams) shiitake mushrooms

2 cups raw walnuts

good bunch flat-leaf parsley

small bunch fresh thyme

2 tablespoons sunflower oil

1 tablespoon olive oil

2 leeks (white part only), finely diced

4 garlic cloves, finely diced

1–2 teaspoons chili flakes (optional)

salt flakes and cracked pepper

16 cannelloni tubes

1. Preheat the oven to 350°F (180°C), and bring a pot of water to a boil.

2. To make the cauliflower béchamel, heat the oil in a large saucepan over medium heat. Add the cauliflower and sprinkle with paprika. Cook for a few minutes, tossing to coat in the oil and get a little flavor happening.

3. Turn up the heat and pour over enough boiling water to completely cover the cauliflower. Season with salt flakes and bring to a simmer. Cook covered on low heat for 25 minutes or until the cauliflower is tender.

4. Remove from the heat and set aside to cool a little before transferring to a food processor or using a stick blender to puree the cauliflower and liquid until smooth.

5. Return to a low heat. Add the milk, nutmeg, nutritional yeast, and cracked pepper, to taste. Bubble gently for a few minute, before adding the lemon juice, to taste.

6. Remove from the heat and set aside. If you want a nice gooey cheesy sauce add around 1–2 cups of vegetarian or nondairy cheese at this stage and stir through. The sauce should be fairly runny as you want a nice amount of liquid to cook the cannelloni—it will thicken as it cooks in the oven.

7. While the cauliflower is cooking you can prepare the mushrooms.

8. Using a food processor, pulse the mushrooms in small batches to obtain a coarse texture. Make sure not to process them too fine, or they will disappear once cooked. Transfer the processed mushrooms to a large bowl.

9. In the same food processor add the walnuts and fresh herbs. Process until you have a coarse breadcrumb consistency. Set aside.

10. Heat the oil over medium heat and add the leeks, cooking for a minute or two until soft. Add around a third of the mushroom mixture and continue to cook over a medium heat for a few minutes before adding the remainder of the mushrooms in two more batches.

11. Toss over medium heat until the mushrooms are tender. Add the garlic and chili flakes, if using, and cook for a few more minutes.

12. Add the processed walnuts and herbs to the mushrooms and stir through, adding salt flakes and generous cracked pepper to taste.

13. Remove from the heat and set aside until the mixture is cool enough to handle. You can transfer it to a large bowl to speed up the process.

14. To assemble the cannelloni, spoon half the cauliflower béchamel into a large baking dish approximately 9 x 12-inches (20 x 30-centimeters) in size.

15. Fill a piping bag (or a sturdy plastic bag like a Ziploc bag with a small hole cut in the corner) with the cooled mushroom mixture.

16. Fill the cannelloni tubes with the mushroom mixture and arrange in the baking dish, side by side, to form one layer. Top the arranged cannelloni tubes with the remaining cauliflower béchamel and sprinkle a little (or a lot) of vegetarian or nondairy cheese over them.

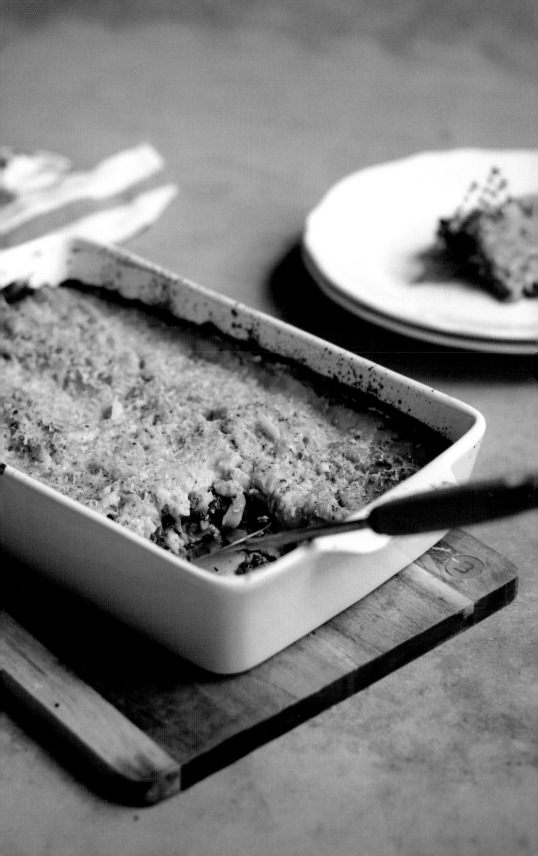

17. Place in the preheated oven for 50 minutes until the top is golden, the sauce is bubbling, and the pasta is tender. Remove from the oven and let it stand for few minutes before serving.

18. Accompany with steamed greens or a crisp salad.

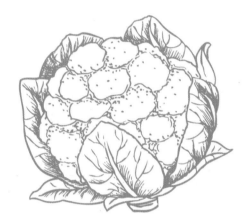

Fragrant Brown Rice and Puy Lentils with Grilled Vegetables and Pine Nut Cream

PREP TIME: 45 MINUTES • SERVES: 4

For added nutritional value try one of the many varieties of rice and grain combinations now readily available in place of the brown rice. Look for those with quinoa, barley, and buckwheat.

WHOLE-GRAIN GOODNESS • PACKED WITH VEGGIE POWER • LEGUME PROTEIN • DIFFICULTY LEVEL **

PINE NUT CREAM

1 cup pine nuts

2 tablespoons olive oil

2 tablespoons lemon juice

salt flakes and cracked pepper, to taste

tiny drizzle of honey or agave nectar, to taste

GRILLED VEGETABLES

2–3 zucchinis

2–3 Japanese eggplants

2 garlic cloves, minced

1 tablespoon olive oil

small bunch fresh sage leaves, torn

salt flakes and cracked pepper

1 tablespoon sunflower oil, for grilling

FRAGRANT BROWN RICE AND PUY LENTILS

½ cup puy lentils (French lentils), rinsed

1 cup brown rice

1 tablespoon sunflower oil

½ red onion, finely diced

1 teaspoon garam masala

1 teaspoon ground turmeric

½ teaspoon ground cinnamon

5 Turkish apricots, diced

1 tablespoon olive oil

zest and juice from 1 lemon

4 cups baby spinach leaves

salt flakes and cracked pepper

fresh lemon wedges, for garnish

1. Place the pine nuts in a small bowl and pour enough water over them to cover. Set aside for at least 10 minutes.

2. To prepare the vegetables, slice the zucchini and eggplant into strips around ⅓-inch (1-centimeter) thick. Toss in a large shallow bowl with the minced garlic, olive oil, and torn sage leaves, adding salt flakes and cracked pepper to taste. Cover and set aside for at least 10 minutes (the vegetables can be prepared like this ahead of time and kept in the fridge for up to 24 hours before grilling).

3. Bring 1½ cups of water to a boil in a saucepan. Add the lentils and turn down the heat to gently simmer, covered, for 25 minutes until the lentils are tender and the water has absorbed. Set aside.

4. Cook the rice according to the packet instructions.

5. Meanwhile make the pine nut cream. Strain off any excess liquid from the pine nuts and add these along with the olive oil, lemon juice, and around 2 tablespoons of water to a blender or small food processor. Blend until the nuts are smooth, adding more water to reach the desired consistency. Add salt flakes, cracked pepper, and a tiny drizzle of honey or agave nectar to taste and whiz again to combine. Set aside.

6. To finish the rice and lentils, heat the sunflower oil in a heavy frying pan over medium heat. Add the diced onion and fry for 3–4 minutes until soft. Add the ground spices and continue to cook over medium-low heat, until the spices are fragrant.

7. Turn up the heat a little and add the cooked lentils and rice, tossing to combine over medium heat. Add the diced apricots and lemon zest and toss again to heat through.

8. Remove from the heat and toss through the olive oil, lemon juice, and baby spinach leaves, adding salt flakes and cracked pepper to taste. Cover and keep warm while you grill the vegetables.

9. To grill the vegetables, heat the sunflower oil in a stovetop grill pan or griddle. Working with a few strips of vegetables at a time, grill over medium-high heat until golden on both sides. Set aside and keep warm on paper towels while you cook the remainder.

10. Serve the grilled vegetables layered over the rice and lentils with dollops of pine nut cream and fresh lemon wedges to serve.

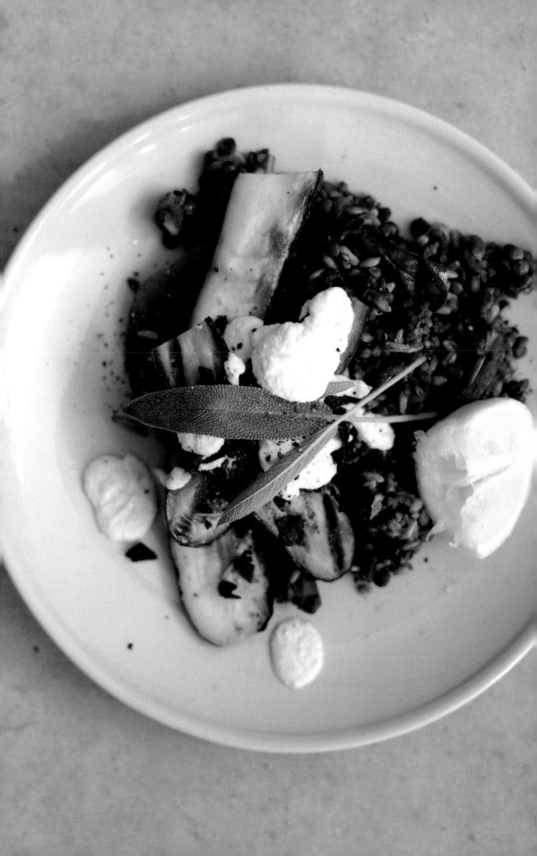

Baked Risotto with Tossed Green Vegetables

PREP TIME: 45 MINUTES • SERVES: 4

Baked risotto is the essence of hassle-free cooking. Prepare the green veggies within the last 10 minutes of the baked risotto cooking time. Use your favorite in-season green vegetables here. Snow peas, snap peas, edamame, kale, and spinach would all work well.

PERFECT FOR NEW VEGETARIANS • PACKED WITH
VEGGIE POWER • DIFFICULTY LEVEL *

BAKED RISOTTO

1 cup arborio rice

2½ cups vegetable stock

juice from 1 orange

TOSSED GREEN VEGETABLES

⅓ cup vegetable stock

juice and zest from 1 orange

1 teaspoon Dijon mustard

2.5 ounces (70 grams) raw almonds, roughly chopped

9 ounces (250 grams) green beans, topped and tailed

1 bunch asparagus, woody ends removed

1 tablespoon olive oil

2 cups baby spinach

1. Preheat the oven to 350°F (180°C).

2. Place the arborio rice, stock, and orange juice in a baking dish and stir to combine. Cover with a tight-fitting lid or with foil and bake in the preheated oven for 40–45 minutes until nearly all liquid is absorbed and rice is al dente.

3. Whisk the stock, orange juice, and Dijon mustard for the vegetables in a small jug or bowl until smooth, and set aside.

4. To prepare the green vegetables, heat a good-sized frying pan or wok and add the almonds. Dry roast, tossing continually, over a medium heat for 1–2 minutes until just brown.

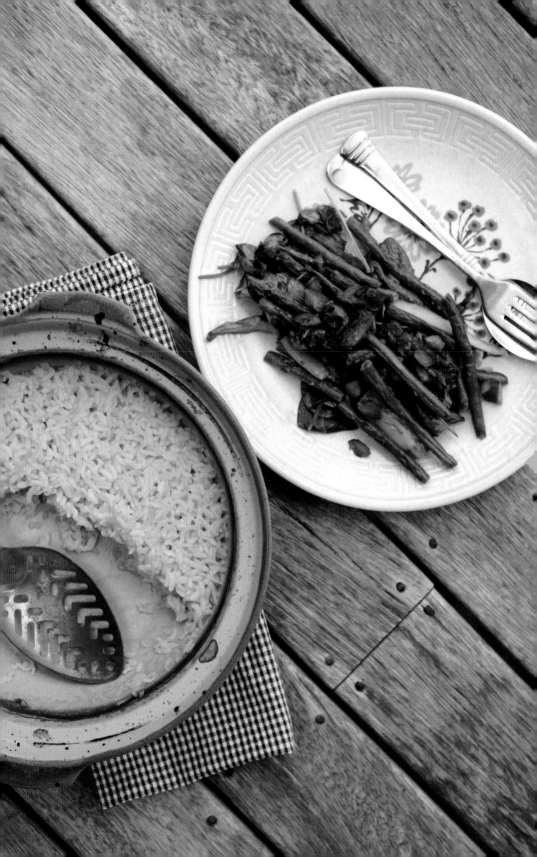

5. Add the beans and asparagus and drizzle with olive oil, tossing in the pan to coat with oil. Increase the heat, adding the stock, mustard, and orange juice mixture and cooking for 2–3 minutes.

6. Add the orange zest and spinach and cook for another minute or until the spinach is just wilted.

7. Serve immediately accompanied by spoonfuls of warm baked risotto.

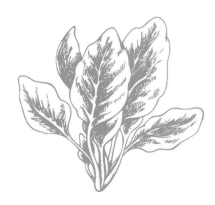

Dal Kofta Balls and Curry

PREP TIME: 80 MINUTES • SERVES: 4–6 AS A MAIN OR 8
AS AN APPETIZER (MAKES 25 KOFTA BALLS)

This kofta takes a little time and effort to prepare, but the amazing flavors of the dish are well worth it. The kofta can be prepared ahead of time and kept covered in the refrigerator; simply pop in the oven to cook while you prepare the curry. Use your favorite good-quality curry paste in this recipe—anything from vindaloo, korma, tandoori, or madras. For something different try serving the kofta balls as an appetizer with the Tofu-tzatziki.

PERFECT FOR NEW VEGETARIANS • LEGUME PROTEIN •
GREAT FOR ENTERTAINING • DIFFICULTY LEVEL ***

DAL KOFTA BALLS

3 cups water

1½ cups red lentils, rinsed

4½ ounces (125 grams) raw cashew nuts

1 yellow onion, finely minced

1 cup whole-grain breadcrumbs

3 teaspoons curry paste

peanut oil, as needed

3 tablespoons golden raisins

DAL KOFTA CURRY

2 tablespoons peanut oil

1 teaspoon mustard seeds

1 teaspoon garam masala

1 teaspoon ground cumin

1 teaspoon ground coriander

½ teaspoon paprika

¼ teaspoon cayenne pepper

2 garlic cloves, minced

2 teaspoons minced fresh ginger

1½ cups vegetable stock

1 (14-ounce/400-gram) can tomato puree

7 ounces (200 milliliters) coconut milk

juice from 1 lime

1 bunch cilantro

TO SERVE

steamed basmati rice

Tofu-tzatziki (page 82)

chutney or lime pickle

1. Preheat the oven to 350°F (180°C) and line two good-sized baking trays with baking paper.

2. Bring the water to a boil in a good-sized saucepan, add the lentils, and reduce the heat to gently simmer, covered, for 25 minutes until lentils are tender and liquid absorbed. Transfer to a large bowl and allow to cool.

3. Using a food processor (or by hand), roughly grind the cashew nuts to a coarse texture. And the ground cashew nuts, along with the minced onion, breadcrumbs, and curry paste to the cooled lentils and combine well.

4. The mixture should come together nicely, a little like cookie dough. Add a little more breadcrumbs if the mixture is too wet or a little peanut oil if the mixture is too dry.

5. Roll a tablespoon of mixture into a ball, placing a golden raisin in the middle of each, and repeat. Arrange the kofta balls on the prepared baking sheets.

6. Place the kofta balls into the preheated oven and cook for 40 minutes, checking after 20 minutes to turn them over.

7. Once lightly golden, remove from the oven and set aside.

8. To prepare the curry, heat the peanut oil in a large heavy frying pan over a medium heat. Add the mustard seeds and heat in the pan for 30 seconds until they begin to pop. Add the ground spices and fry over a low heat to form a paste, then add the garlic and ginger and continue to cook for another minute.

9. Add the stock and tomato puree and bring to a gentle simmer for 5 minutes until reduced slightly. Gently add the roasted kofta balls and cook for another 3–4 minutes, moving the kofta balls around carefully as they may begin to break up a little. This adds to the texture and thickness of the curry sauce, so don't be too alarmed. Just be careful to cook them gently so they do stay mostly together.

10. Add the coconut milk a little at a time and continue to gently cook over low heat for another few minutes. Remove from the heat and add a good squeeze or two of lime juice and scatter with freshly torn cilantro before serving immediately.

11. Accompany with plenty of steamed basmati rice, plus the Tofu-tzatziki and chutney or lime pickle, for a complete curry meal.

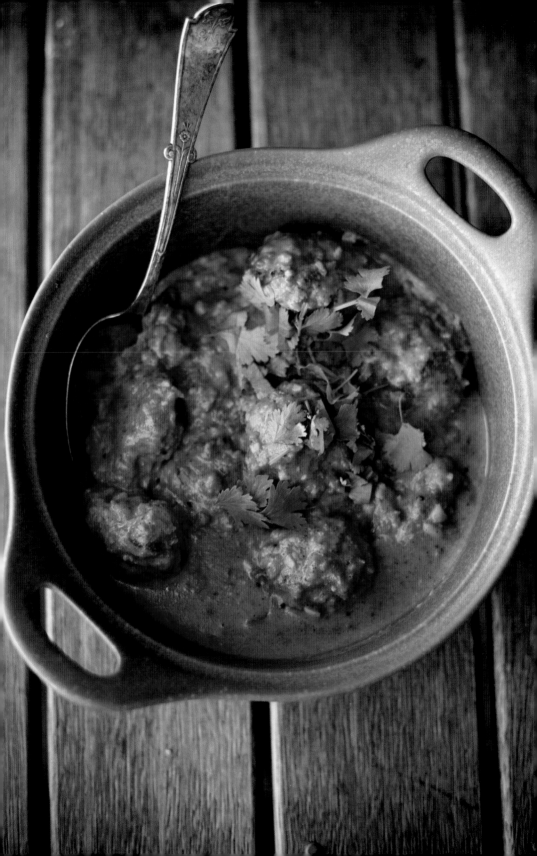

Baked Fennel and Vegetable Medley with Quinoa

PREP TIME: 40 MINUTES • SERVES: 2–4

If you can't find baby carrots, use larger carrots cut into batons.
Either red or white quinoa is lovely in this dish. Buckwheat,
barley, or couscous are great substitutes for the quinoa.

PACKED WITH VEGGIE POWER • WHOLE-GRAIN GOODNESS
• GREAT FOR ENTERTAINING • DIFFICULTY LEVEL *

---

6 ounces (175 grams) baby carrots, scrubbed

6 ounces (175 grams) asparagus, woody ends removed

5 ounces (150 grams) patty pan squash, quartered

½ large fennel bulb, sliced

¼ cup olive oil

1 teaspoon salt flakes

½ teaspoon chili flakes (optional)

2–3 star anise

1 cup quinoa

3 cups vegetable stock

1 tablespoon almonds

1 tablespoon hazelnuts

1. Preheat the oven to 400°F (200°C).

2. Toss the vegetables in the olive oil, salt, and chili flakes, if using, making sure all the vegetables are well coated in oil.

3. Arrange the prepared vegetables in a large baking tray and toss in all of the star anise.

4. Roast the vegetables in the preheated oven for 30 minutes until golden and still slightly firm.

5. Meanwhile, bring the quinoa and vegetable stock to a boil in a small saucepan. Turn down the heat and allow to simmer for 15 minutes until tender. Strain off any excess liquid and keep warm until serving.

6. Dry roast the nuts in a frying pan over medium heat and then allow to cool before chopping coarsely.

7. Removing the star anise, toss the baked vegetables with the chopped almonds and hazelnuts and serve on a bed of warm prepared quinoa.

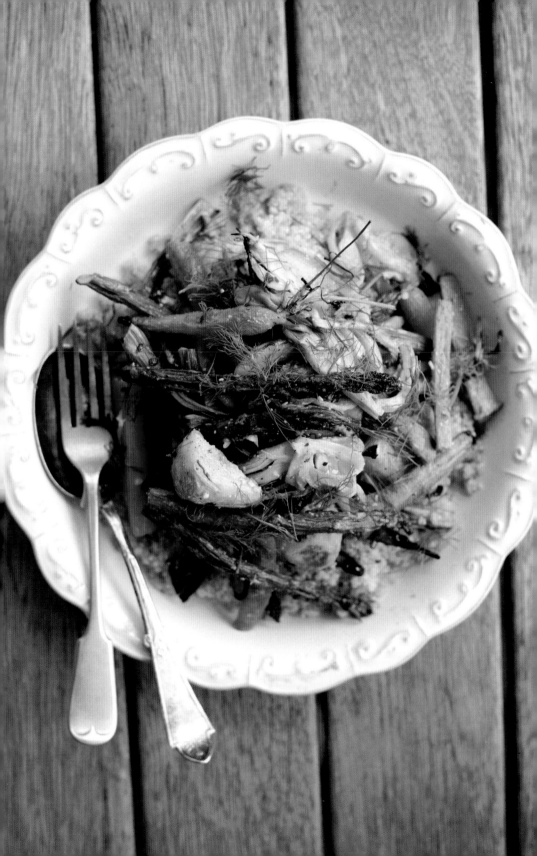

Curried Black Rice Soup with Green Veg and Silken Tofu

PREP TIME: 55 MINUTES • SERVES: 4

If you can't find black rice simply substitute with brown or basmati. You can use your favorite seasonal green vegetables here like Brussels sprouts, broccoli, and asparagus. Or try frozen peas, broccoli, beans, or even spinach when green vegetables are out of season. Curry leaves should be available at your local Asian food store. Try dried curry leaves if you can't find fresh—simply increase the amount.

WHOLE-GRAIN GOODNESS • PACKED WITH VEGGIE POWER • SOY PROTEIN • DIFFICULTY LEVEL: *

¼ cup peanut oil

1 tablespoon mustard seeds

1 small yellow onion, finely diced

2 teaspoons cumin seeds

1 teaspoon garam masala

1 teaspoon paprika

2 teaspoons ground turmeric

small handful of fresh curry leaves

3 garlic cloves, finely diced

1-inch (5-centimeter) piece of fresh ginger, grated

2 red chilies, finely diced (seeds removed if you prefer)

1 teaspoon dark brown sugar

1 cup black rice (or brown or basmati)

1 quart (1 liter) vegetable stock

2 cups water

2 cups snow peas, sliced in half diagonally

1 bunch of broccolini, cut into florets

10 ounces (300 grams) silken tofu, diced into large cubes

TO SERVE

½ English cucumber, grated

1 red chili, finely diced (seeds removed if you prefer)

½ cup fresh grated coconut (or use pre-shredded coconut)

handful of fresh cilantro leaves, roughly torn

1 lime, cut into wedges

1. Heat the peanut oil in a large heavy pot over medium-low heat. Add the mustard seeds and heat gently until they begin to pop. Add the onion and fry over medium-low heat until soft.

2. Add the dry spices and curry leaves, cooking over low heat for a minute or two until fragrant and a paste begins to form. Add the garlic, ginger, chili, and brown sugar, and cook for another minute.

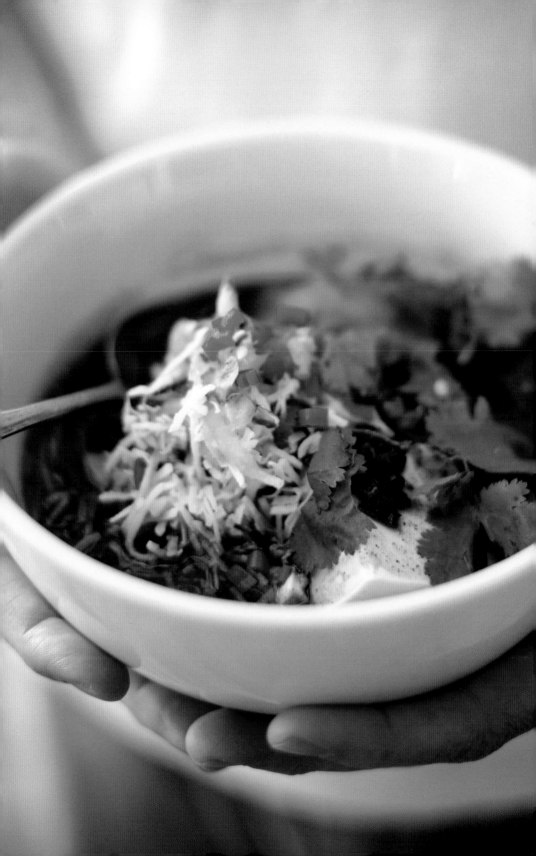

3. Add the rice and toss to combine. Increase the heat and add the stock and water.

4. Bring to a simmer, then reduce heat to very low and gently simmer, covered, for 30–40 minutes until rice is tender. If you're using basmati or brown rice, reduce the cooking time by about 10–15 minutes, or until the rice is tender.

5. Just before serving, pop the snow peas and broccolini into the soup to simmer for only a minute to be sure they do not overcook—you want them to be a little crunchy.

6. To serve, ladle the soup into large bowls over cubes of silken tofu and top with the grated cucumber, coconut, cilantro, and chili to taste, adding a squeeze of lime.

Soda-Battered Eggplant with Carrot Chips, Sprout Salad, and Fresh Pickle

PREP TIME: 55 MINUTES • SERVES: 4

The pickle, batter, and sprout salad can all be made ahead of time. The carrot chips and soda-battered eggplant are best served immediately while still hot and crunchy. Make sure to get your oil nice and hot before adding the strips of battered eggplant and fry only one or two pieces at a time for the best results.

PERFECT FOR NEW VEGETARIANS • PACKED WITH VEGGIE POWER • GREAT FOR ENTERTAINING • DIFFICULTY LEVEL ***

FRESH CUCUMBER PICKLE

1 Persian cucumber

1 lemon

1 tablespoon olive oil

½ teaspoon dill seeds

SODA-BATTERED EGGPLANT

1 cup all-purpose flour

1½ teaspoons baking powder

½ teaspoon ground turmeric

2 teaspoons nutritional yeast

1 cup chilled soda water (sparkling water)

3–4 Japanese eggplants

salt

peanut or sunflower oil, for deep-frying

CARROT CHIPS

4 large carrots, diced into ½-centimeter rounds (approximately 4 cups)

2 tablespoons olive oil

small bunch fresh thyme

salt flakes and cracked pepper

SPROUT SALAD

2 cups snow pea sprouts

2 cups bean sprouts

1 cup legume sprouts (mung, chickpea, lentil)

1½ tablespoons lemon juice

3 tablespoons olive oil

tiny drizzle of honey or agave nectar

salt flakes and cracked pepper

1. Preheat the oven to 400°F (200°C).

2. First, prepare the pickle by slicing the cucumber in half lengthways and then very thinly slicing. Also slice the lemon in half lengthways before seeding and finely dicing one half (reserving the other half for use later).

3. Heat the olive oil in a small saucepan over medium-low heat. Add the dill seeds and continue to heat until they begin to pop and crackle. Add the prepared cucumber and lemon and toss over medium heat for just 1 minute.

4. Remove from the heat and squeeze over the juice of the remaining half a lemon. Set aside to cool before placing in the refrigerator to chill.

5. Prepare the soda batter by sifting the flour and baking powder into a big mixing bowl. Add the turmeric and nutritional yeast and stir to combine. Pour over the soda water and whisk until smooth. Pop in the fridge and chill while you prepare the sprout salad and carrot chips.

6. Place two good-sized baking trays in the oven to preheat for 3–4 minutes.

7. Carefully remove the preheated trays from the oven and line with baking paper. Arrange the rounds of carrot in a single layer over the two baking trays. Drizzle with olive oil and sprinkle fresh thyme on top and with salt flakes and cracked pepper, to taste.

8. Place in the hot oven, roasting for 30 minutes until the carrots are golden and crisp.

9. Slice the eggplants lengthways into strips around ½ inch (1.5 centimeters) thick. Place the eggplant strips onto paper towels and sprinkle over a few pinches of salt flakes. Leave for a few minutes until the eggplants begin to sweat. Turn over and repeat on the other side, patting the eggplant strips dry after a few more minutes and pricking the skins with a fork.

10. Meanwhile, prepare the sprout salad by roughly dicing the tops of the snow pea sprouts and finely dicing the stalks. Add these along with the bean and legume sprouts to a large serving bowl. Toss with your hands to combine.

11. Make the sprout salad dressing by adding all the lemon juice, olive oil, and honey or agave nectar, with salt flakes and cracked pepper to taste, to a screw top jar and shaking until well combined. Place both the salad and dressing into the refrigerator until ready to serve.

12. To deep-fry the eggplant, pour your oil into a good-sized deep pot up to a depth of around 6 inches (15 centimeters) and heat on high until the surface begins to shimmer.

13. Remove the batter from the refrigerator and whisk again, quickly, until smooth. Working with one piece at a time, dip a strip of prepared eggplant into the batter. Allow the excess to drip off before carefully sliding into the hot oil.

14. The batter should quickly begin to sizzle and golden. Fry for 1 minute before turning to fry on the other side for just 1 more minute. Remove with a slotted ladle and place on paper towels. Keep warm while you deep-fry the remaining pieces.

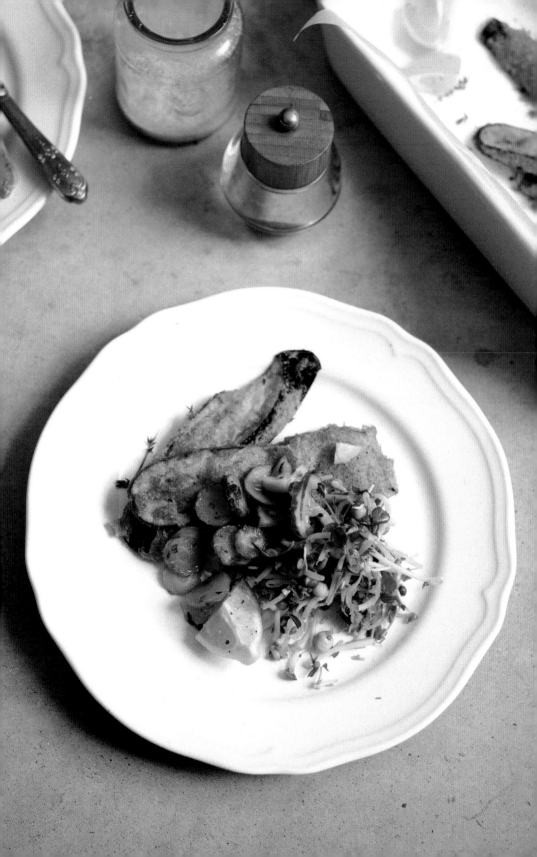

15. Just before serving, pour any excess liquid off the pickles and place in a serving dish. Shake the sprout salad dressing again and then pour over the sprouts, tossing to combine.

16. Serve the warm soda-battered eggplant and hot carrot chips accompanied by the sprout salad and fresh pickle.

FAMILY MEALS

Fragrant Couscous with Veg Sausage, Chickpeas, Almonds, and Apricots

PREP TIME: 25 MINUTES • SERVES: 4

Use your favorite vegetarian soy or chickpea sausage or try grilled mushrooms or roasted pumpkin instead. If you enjoy dairy, a little vegetarian feta is nice tossed in at the end.

PERFECT FOR NEW VEGETARIANS • WHOLE-GRAIN GOODNESS • KID-APPROVED • DIFFICULTY LEVEL *

2 cups vegetable stock, divided

1½ cups whole wheat couscous

1 tablespoon sunflower oil, divided

10 ounces (300 grams) vegetarian sausages

2 tablespoons olive oil, divided

1 teaspoon ground turmeric

1 teaspoon smoked paprika

½ teaspoon ground cardamom

¼ teaspoon cayenne pepper (optional)

2 garlic cloves, finely minced

2 cups chickpeas (cooked or canned)

¼ cup dry roasted almonds, roughly chopped

¼ cup dried Turkish apricots, diced

¼ cup fresh mint, roughly chopped

zest and juice from 1 lemon

salt flakes and cracked pepper

1. Bring 1½ cups of the stock to boil in a small saucepan. Remove from the heat and pour in the couscous. Cover and set aside for 5 minutes until the liquid is absorbed.

2. Fluff the couscous with a fork to separate the grains; cover again and keep warm while you prepare the remainder of the ingredients.

3. Heat half the sunflower oil in a heavy frying pan and cook the sausages on medium heat, turning frequently until golden. Remove from the heat and slice diagonally, then set aside.

4. Add half a tablespoon of the olive oil with the remainder of the sunflower oil to the same pan and over medium-low heat, add the spices, and cook gently for 1 minute until fragrant and a smooth paste forms. Add the garlic and fry gently for another minute.

5. Increase the heat and add the chickpeas plus a splash or two of the remaining stock. Cook off the liquid over medium heat for 2–3 minutes before adding the sliced sausage, almonds, and apricots. Toss to combine and remove from the heat.

6. Combine the sausage and chickpea mixture with the prepared couscous, and dress with the mint, lemon juice, and remaining olive oil. Season with salt flakes and fresh cracked pepper, to taste, and toss well.

7. Serve warm with a side of Tossed Green Vegetables (page 122) or with thick slices of dark rye bread spread with hummus.

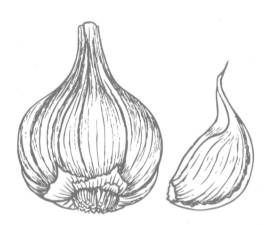

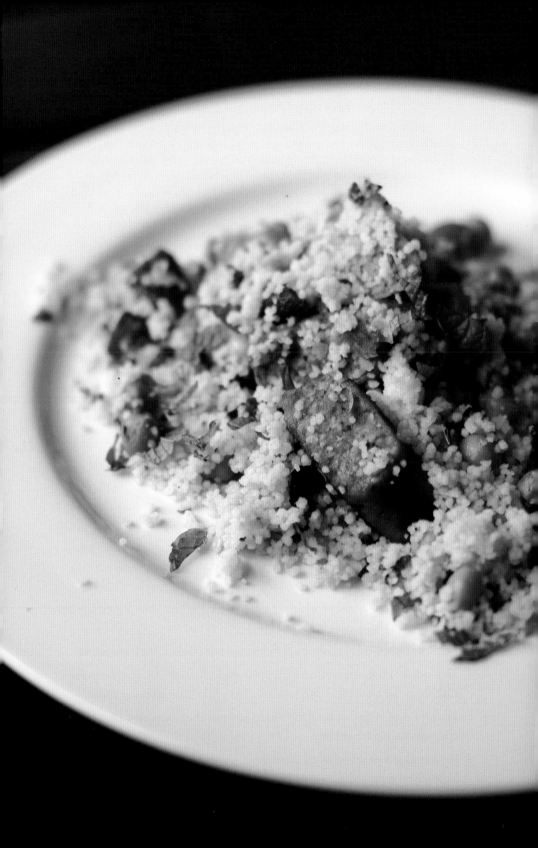

Tempeh Pot Pies

PREP TIME: 60 MINUTES • SERVES: 4

You can use this recipe to make one large pie, rather than smaller pot pies. Lacto-vegetarians can replace the soy milk and cream with dairy, if preferred. Check the listed ingredients on the filo pastry you buy, or go for one that clearly states suitable for vegetarians or vegan-friendly.

> PERFECT FOR NEW VEGETARIANS • KID-APPROVED • GREAT FOR ENTERTAINING • SOY PROTEIN • DIFFICULTY LEVEL **

9 ounces (250 grams) tempeh	1 tablespoons whole wheat flour
3 tablespoons cornstarch	1 cup vegetable stock
3 tablespoons sunflower oil, divided	½ tablespoon Dijon mustard, or to taste
2 large leeks, diced	1 cup peas
3 young carrots, diced	⅓ cup soy cream
7 ounces (200 grams) button mushrooms, diced	8 sheets of filo pastry
	¼ cup soy milk

1. Preheat the oven to 400°F (200°C).

2. Tear the tempeh into chunks and toss lightly in the cornstarch. Heat 2 tablespoons of the sunflower oil in a heavy frying pan and fry the tempeh in batches over medium heat until lightly golden. Place on paper towels and set aside.

3. Heat the remaining oil in the same pan and fry the leeks and carrots over a medium heat for 3–4 minutes until the leeks are soft. Add the mushrooms and continue to cook for another 3–4 minutes until the mushrooms start to soften.

4. Add the whole wheat flour and cook for 2–3 minutes, gradually adding the stock and stirring to combine; add the mustard and cook for another 3–4 minutes.

5. Remove from the heat and add the prepared tempeh, peas, and soy cream. Stir to combine well.

6. Place the ingredients into four lightly greased ramekins or one large pie dish.

7. Top with 4 or 5 sheets of filo pastry, brushing with a little soy milk between each sheet. Trim the edges and brush the top with a little extra soy milk.

8. Place the pies in the hot oven for 30–35 minutes until the pastry is golden and crisp and the pie is bubbling.

9. Serve hot, accompanied by steamed green vegetables, or try the Tossed Green Vegetables on page 122.

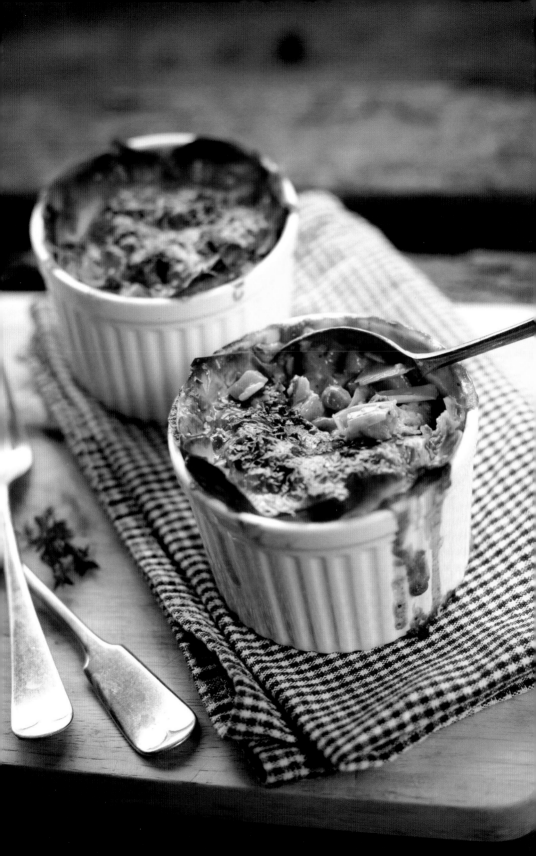

Buckwheat, Mushroom, and Rye Burgers with Quick Tomato Relish and Kale Chips

PREP TIME: 50 MINUTES, SERVES: 6–12

Use your favorite burger buns here and add any extras, such as pickles, grilled pineapple, sprouts, and nondairy or dairy cheese. The tomato relish and burger patty mixture can be prepared the day before and kept covered in the refrigerator. This recipe makes 12 small or 6 large patties.

PERFECT FOR NEW VEGETARIANS • PACKED WITH VEGGIE POWER • WHOLE-GRAIN GOODNESS • GREAT FOR ENTERTAINING • KID-APPROVED • DIFFICULTY LEVEL **

BUCKWHEAT, MUSHROOM, AND RYE BURGER PATTIES

½ cup raw buckwheat

1–2 slices seeded whole-grain bread

1 cup rolled rye or oats

2 cups button mushrooms, quartered

1 yellow onion

small bunch of flat-leaf parsley

small bunch fresh thyme leaves

2 tablespoons nutritional yeast

1 tablespoon Dijon mustard, or to taste

2 teaspoons balsamic vinegar

1–2 teaspoons chili flakes (optional)

salt flakes and cracked pepper

KALE CHIPS

1 large bunch kale

1–2 tablespoons olive oil

2 teaspoons nutritional yeast

salt flakes

ADDITIONAL INGREDIENTS

1–2 tablespoons sunflower oil

6–12 burger buns, lightly toasted

soy or traditional mayonnaise

crisp lettuce leaves

sliced tomato

sliced cucumber

Quick Tomato Relish (page 80)

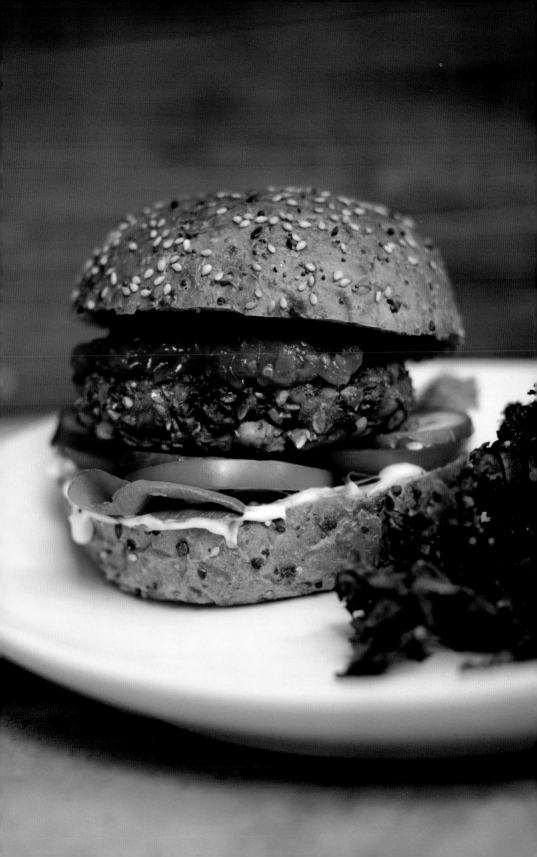

1. Bring the buckwheat and 1½ cups of water to a boil in a saucepan. Gently simmer, covered, over low heat for 30 minutes, or until liquid is absorbed and the buckwheat is tender. Set aside to cool.

2. Place the slices of bread in a food processor and process until you have coarse breadcrumbs; set aside in a separate small bowl.

3. Add the rolled rye or oats to the same food processor and process to a coarse flour. Transfer to a large bowl.

4. Place the chopped mushrooms in the same food processor and process until you have a ground meat consistency. Transfer to the same bowl as the prepared rolled rye.

5. Process the onion with the fresh parsley and thyme until finely minced. Transfer to the mushrooms and rye. Add the cooled buckwheat, nutritional yeast, mustard, balsamic vinegar, and chili flakes, if using, with salt flakes and generous cracked pepper, to taste.

6. Using your hands, combine all the ingredients, adding the prepared breadcrumbs a little at a time until you have a good burger patty mixture that's not too wet and holds together nicely. Set aside, covered, in the refrigerator until you are ready to grill.

7. To make the kale chips, preheat the oven to 350°F (180°C) and line two large baking trays with baking paper.

8. Trim the steams off the kale leaves and tear into bite-size pieces.

9. Lay the kale pieces over the two baking trays, drizzle with the olive oil, and sprinkle over with the nutritional yeast. Toss briefly to combine and then place in a preheated oven for 10–15 minutes, until crisp. Remove from the oven and serve sprinkled with salt flakes.

10. To grill the burger patties, heat a small amount of the sunflower oil on a stovetop or barbecue grill pan. Once hot, roll portions of the patty mixture into balls and drop onto the grill. Use the back of a spatula to flatten down the patties and grill over medium-high heat for a few minutes, turning to grill on the other side until golden and crunchy on the outside. Set aside on paper towels while you grill the remainder.

11. To make the burgers, spread the bottom half of the toasted bun with your choice of mayonnaise. Top with lettuce leaves, tomato, cucumber, a burger patty, and a good dollop or two of the tomato relish. Serve burgers accompanied with kale chips.

Lentil Bolognese Lasagna

PREP TIME: 55 MINUTES • SERVES: 6

This recipe makes a delicious, hearty meal, sure to satisfy even the most devout meat-eater. Use your favorite nondairy butter and cheese. Or, those who aren't strict vegetarians can replace the butter, cheese, and milk with dairy.

> PERFECT FOR NEW VEGETARIANS • KID-APPROVED • GREAT FOR ENTERTAINING • LEGUME PROTEIN • DIFFICULTY LEVEL **

1 ½ cups brown lentils, rinsed

4 cups vegetable stock, divided

3 bay leaves

2 tablespoons sunflower oil

2 teaspoons olive oil

1 yellow onion, diced

2 garlic cloves, diced

1 large carrot, grated

9 ounces (250 grams) cherry tomatoes, halved

2 tablespoons balsamic vinegar

1 teaspoon raw sugar

½ cup tomato paste

salt flakes and cracked pepper, to taste

WHITE SAUCE

2 ounces (50 grams) nondairy butter

¼ cup whole wheat flour

12 fluid ounces (350 milliliters) soy or oat milk

½ teaspoon ground nutmeg

salt flakes and cracked pepper

8 lasagna sheets

½ cup grated nondairy or vegetarian sharp cheddar or pecorino cheese

1. Bring 3 cups of the stock and the bay leaves to a boil in a large saucepan. Add the lentils, turn down the heat, and simmer, covered, for 20 minutes. Remove from the heat.

2. Preheat the oven to 400°F (200°C).

3. While the lentils are simmering, heat the sunflower and olive oil in a large frying pan. Add the onion and cook over medium heat until soft.

4. Add the garlic and cook for another minute until fragrant. Add the carrot and cherry tomatoes, with the balsamic vinegar. Fry for 1 minute before adding the remaining 1 cup of stock, sugar, and tomato paste, and simmer over low heat for a few minutes.

5. Add the lentils and any remaining cooking liquid and continue to simmer for 10–15 minutes; season with salt flakes and cracked pepper, to taste.

6. To make the white sauce, melt the butter in a medium saucepan over low heat; add in the flour, stirring with a wooden spoon for around 1 minute until combined. Remove from the heat and gradually add the milk, whisking until smooth.

7. Return to the heat and slowly bring to a gentle boil, stirring over a low heat for 5 minutes until sauce starts to thicken. Remove from the heat, stir in the nutmeg, and season with salt flakes and cracked pepper to taste. Set aside.

8. In a large baking dish, spoon in a layer of the lentils, spread with a layer of white sauce, and then top with a single layer of lasagna sheets. Repeat with more layers, finishing with lentils and white sauce. Sprinkle cheese evenly over the top and bake in the preheated oven for 30–35 minutes until golden on top.

9. Serve with a simple green salad.

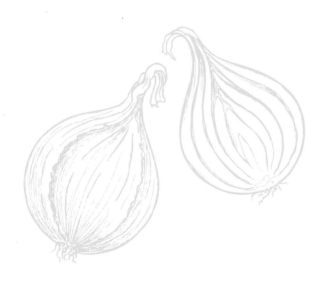

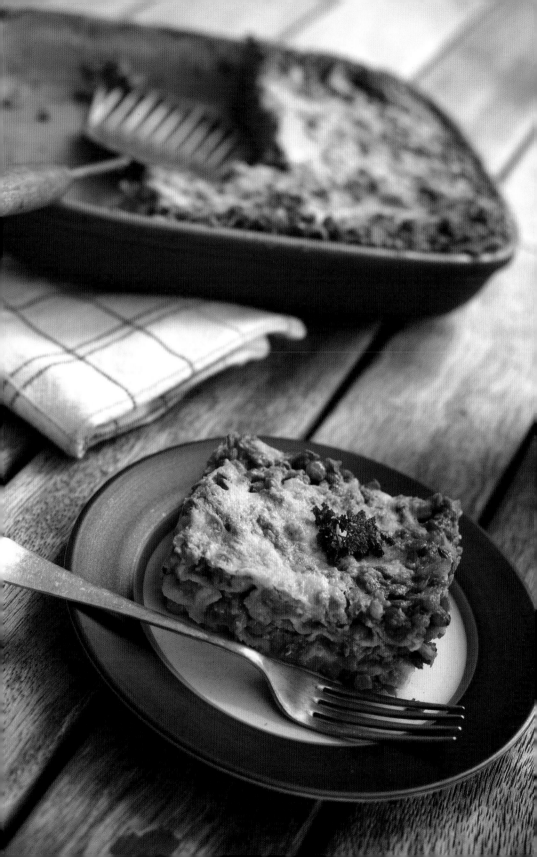

Curried Lentil Soup with Coconut and Cashews

PREP TIME: 40 MINUTES • SERVES: 4

You can substitute ground cumin here for the cumin seeds to save time. This recipe makes a lovely meal on its own, or a hearty dinner served with the rice and pappadams or naan bread.

> PERFECT FOR NEW VEGETARIANS • KID-APPROVED
> • LEGUME PROTEIN • DIFFICULTY LEVEL *

2 teaspoons cumin seeds

2 tablespoons peanut or sunflower oil

1 teaspoon mustard seeds

1 yellow onion, finely diced

1 teaspoon garam masala

1 teaspoon minced fresh or ground turmeric

2 garlic cloves, minced

2 teaspoons minced fresh ginger

1 green chili, seeded and finely diced (optional)

1 pound (450 grams) red lentils, rinsed

14 ounces (400 grams) tomatoes, roughly diced

½ teaspoon raw sugar

6 cups vegetable stock

TO SERVE

¼ cup raw cashew nuts, roughly chopped

¼ cup shredded coconut

¼ cup golden raisins

¼ cup fresh cilantro, chopped

Tofu-tzatziki (page 82) (optional)

pappadams or naan bread (optional)

steamed basmati rice (optional)

1. Dry roast the cumin seeds in a heavy pot or deep-frying pan over medium heat for around 2 minutes, tossing frequently, until fragrant. Remove from the pan and grind the seeds finely.

2. In the same pot or pan, heat the oil and the mustard seeds over high heat until the seeds start to pop. Add the onion and fry over medium heat until soft. Turn down the heat a little, add the spices, including the dry roasted and ground cumin plus the garlic, ginger, and chili, if using, and continue to cook over medium-low heat for another minute, until fragrant.

3. Add the red lentils and toss to combine. Add the chopped tomatoes and sprinkle with the sugar. Bring the heat up to medium-high and add a splash of stock, continuing to toss the tomatoes and lentils with the spice mixture for a minute or so, adding more stock when needed to stop it from sticking.

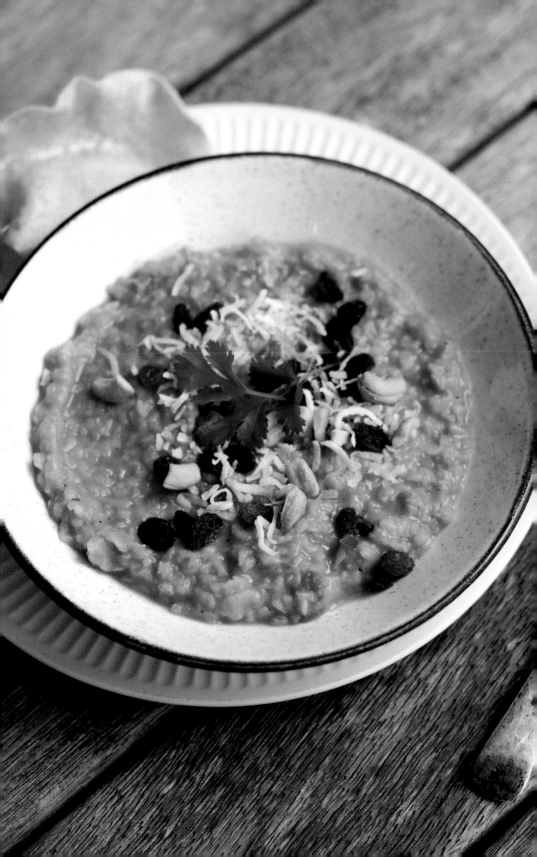

4. Add the remaining stock and bring to a gentle simmer. Cook uncovered for 25 minutes, until lentils are soft and the soup is a thick stew.

5. Serve in warm bowls topped with chopped cashew nuts, shredded coconut, raisins, and fresh cilantro, accompanied with Tofu-tzatziki, pappadams, or naan bread, and steamed basmati rice, if you wish.

Sweet Potato and Kale Quesadillas

Replace the kale with spinach if you prefer. If using soy cheese, go for one that melts well, as this will help hold the quesadilla together. Any tortillas or flat bread should work well—try corn or whole wheat tortillas, or even seeded or whole-grain wraps. These quesadillas go particularly well with the Sprout Salad on page 133.

> PERFECT FOR NEW VEGETARIANS • KID-APPROVED • PACKED WITH VEGGIE POWER • GREAT FOR ENTERTAINING • DIFFICULTY LEVEL **

CUMIN ROASTED SWEET POTATO

1 pound (450 grams) sweet potato, scrubbed and cubed

2 tablespoons olive oil

1 teaspoon honey or maple syrup

2 teaspoons ground cumin

1 teaspoon ground cinnamon

salt flakes and cracked pepper, to coat

CORN AND RED BEANS

2 tablespoons sunflower oil

1 red onion, peeled and finely diced

1–2 teaspoon smoked paprika

½ teaspoon ground cinnamon

2 garlic cloves, crushed

1½ cups corn kernels (approximately 2 cobs of corn)

1½ cups red kidney beans, cooked or canned (equivalent to a 15-ounce can)

good handful of fresh cilantro, roughly chopped

juice from 1 lime

ADDITIONAL INGREDIENTS

4 ounces (120 grams) kale

8 tortillas

1–2 cups grated cheese (nondairy or dairy)

1 tablespoon sunflower oil, for cooking

1 lime (optional)

1. Preheat the oven to 350°F (180°C).

2. Throw the cubed sweet potato into a baking dish. Drizzle with the olive oil, honey or maple syrup, and spices. Toss to evenly coat the cubes and sprinkle on a little ground salt flakes and cracked pepper.

3. Place in the preheated oven for 20–25 minutes, until soft and golden.

4. Meanwhile, heat the sunflower oil in a good-sized frying pan over medium heat. Add the onion and fry for a few minutes until soft. Add the spices

and fry over medium-low heat until fragrant, then add the garlic and fry for another minute.

5. Increase the heat and add the corn kernels and beans. Toss together over a medium heat for 10–15 minutes, or until the corn kernels start to turn golden and the beans begin to stick a little.

6. Once the sweet potato pieces are ready, transfer them to the frying pan with the corn and beans and toss to combine well, squashing everything down a little. Remove from the heat and toss in the chopped cilantro, squeezing the lime juice on top. Set aside.

7. Roughly chop the kale and place in a deep bowl. Pour over with enough hot water to cover and blanch for 30 seconds before draining and rinsing under cold water. Set aside.

8. To assemble the quesadillas, arrange 4 tortillas on a clean surface. Sprinkle each with a little cheese, evenly distribute the blanched kale, and then top with a few spoonfuls of the sweet potato and corn mixture. Add a little extra cheese and finish by topping with the remaining tortillas.

9. To cook the quesadillas, brush a small amount of oil over the bottom of a heavy frying pan (or a grill or griddle). Working with one at a time, carefully place the assembled quesadilla into the hot pan and fry for a minute or two until golden, and then carefully flip to cook on the other side.

10. The quesadillas are ready once crisp and golden on the outside and melted and hot through the middle. Transfer the cooked quesadilla onto paper towels and keep covered and warm while you cook the remainder.

11. Cut the cooked quesadillas into four and serve with wedges of lime and salad of your choice.

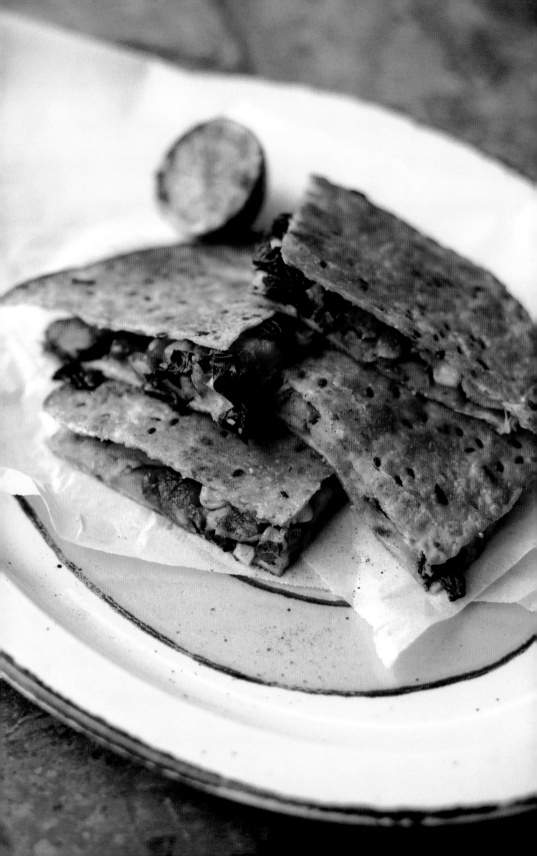

Roasted Pumpkin and Sage Spelt Pasta with Pumpkin Seed and Spinach Pesto

PREP TIME: 45 MINUTES • SERVES: 4

The pumpkin seed and spinach pesto is great served on sandwiches, in wraps, or with crackers for dipping. You can roast the garlic for the pesto along with the pumpkin for a milder flavor. This dish makes a lovely light meal; add vegetarian sausage for a little more substance and protein. Those who enjoy dairy can try a little vegetarian feta cheese tossed in at the end.

PACKED WITH VEGGIE POWER • WHOLE-GRAIN GOODNESS
• KID-APPROVED • DIFFICULTY LEVEL *

PUMPKIN SEED AND SPINACH PESTO

½ cup pumpkin seeds

1½ teaspoons maple syrup

salt flakes and cracked pepper

3 cups spinach

1 garlic clove

¼–½ cup walnut or olive oil

ADDITIONAL INGREDIENTS

3 cups diced pumpkin

1–2 tablespoons olive oil

salt flakes and cracked pepper

bunch of fresh sage

9 ounces (250 grams) spelt pasta

1. To make the pesto, add the pumpkin seeds to a heavy pan and dry roast over medium-low heat until they begin to crackle and pop. Remove from the heat and drizzle the maple syrup on top along with the salt flakes and cracked pepper, to taste. The maple syrup should almost candy when it hits the hot seeds. Allow to cool.

2. Transfer half the pumpkin seed mixture to a food processor, reserving the remainder.

3. Add the spinach and garlic to the food processor. With the motor running gradually add the walnut oil until you have a loose (runny) pesto. Set aside.

4. Preheat the oven to 350°F (180°C).

5. Throw the diced pumpkin into a baking tray and drizzle with the olive oil. Sprinkle on a little pinch of salt flakes and cracked pepper, to taste. Toss well and place in the preheated oven for around 25 minutes.

6. Meanwhile, cook the spelt pasta according to the packet instructions.

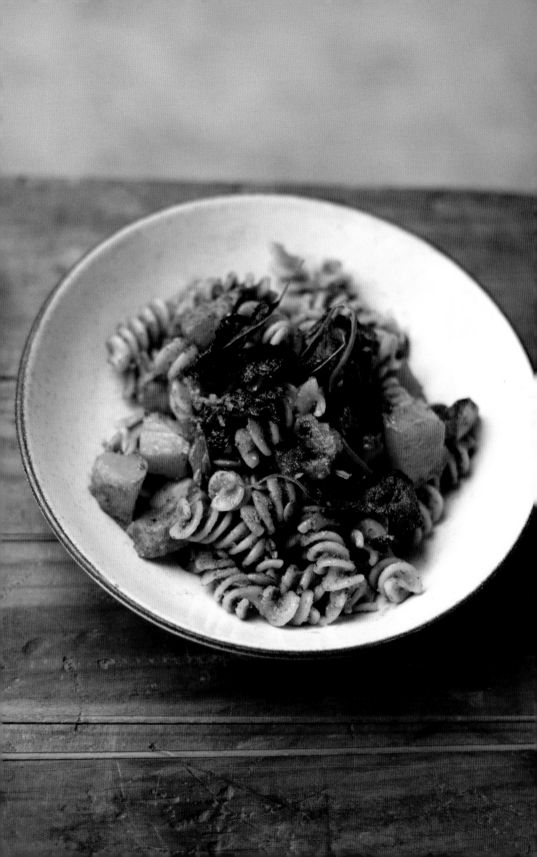

7. When the pumpkin pieces just begin to turn golden on the edges, add the sage leaves and return to the oven for another 5 or so minutes until the pumpkin is soft and golden and the sage leaves are crisp.

8. Add the cooked pasta to the same heavy pan you dry roasted the pumpkin seeds in and toss over medium heat with the prepared pesto until well coated. Add the roasted pumpkin, sage leaves, and reserved pumpkin seeds. Toss gently to combine.

9. Serve warm or, alternatively, prepare ahead of time and serve as a cold pasta salad.

Tofu Tacos with Slaw, Grilled Corn, Chili Cashew Cream, and Roasted Salsa

PREP TIME: 90 MINUTES • SERVES: 4–6

Although nothing is too difficult, there are a few elements to this dish, so allow plenty of time in the kitchen to prepare everything. The roasted salsa, slaw, and cashew cream can be made ahead. Simply reheat the salsa before serving. You can also substitute traditional breadcrumbs for the panko.

> PERFECT FOR NEW VEGETARIANS • KID-APPROVED • PACKED WITH VEGGIE POWER • GREAT FOR ENTERTAINING • SOY PROTEIN • DIFFICULTY LEVEL **

ROASTED SALSA

3 ripe tomatoes

1 red bell pepper

1 red chili (optional)

½ red onion

2 garlic cloves, with skins on

1–2 tablespoons olive oil

1 teaspoon cumin seeds

½ teaspoon fennel seeds

¼ teaspoon brown sugar

1 tablespoon tomato paste

salt flakes and cracked pepper

CHILI CASHEW CREAM

1¼ cups raw cashew nuts

2 tablespoons olive oil

2 tablespoons lime juice

1–2 teaspoons chili sauce (or tomato paste for a mild version)

salt flakes and cracked pepper

SLAW

¼ red cabbage, shredded

1 green apple, grated

2 tablespoons egg-free mayonnaise

1 tablespoon olive oil

1 tablespoon lime juice

¼ teaspoon honey or agave nectar

salt flakes and cracked pepper

GRILLED CORN

3 corn ears

2 teaspoons olive oil

1 teaspoon smoked paprika

1 teaspoon ground cinnamon

1 teaspoon cayenne pepper (optional)

salt flakes and cracked pepper, to taste

juice from 1 lime

small bunch fresh cilantro

BREADED TOFU

2 teaspoons chia seeds

½ cup water

13 ounces (375 grams) firm tofu

1 cup panko crumbs or rice crumbs

1 teaspoon ground cumin

¼ cup whole wheat flour

sunflower or peanut oil, for deep-frying

ADDITIONAL INGREDIENTS

8–10 tortillas

1 avocado, sliced

lime wedges

1. Preheat the oven to 350°F (180°C).

2. Place the cashew nuts for the cashew cream in a bowl with enough water to cover and set aside to soak for around 10–15 minutes.

3. For the roasted salsa, slice the tomatoes, bell pepper, and chili, if using, in half, removing the seeds and membrane from the pepper and chili. Quarter the onion, leaving the skin on.

4. Lay the tomatoes, bell pepper, and chili cut-side down on a baking tray. Throw in the onion wedges and whole garlic cloves, with skins on. Drizzle with the olive oil and sprinkle with the spices. Toss well to coat everything in the oil and spices and then place in the preheated oven.

5. Bake for 25–30 minutes until the tomatoes and bell peppers are blistered and beginning to darken. Remove from the oven and set aside to cool.

6. Once cool, peel and discard the tomato, bell pepper, and onion skins, and squash the garlic from their skins. Add all the ingredients from the roasting pan, including the juices and oil in the bottom, a food processor. Add the brown sugar and tomato paste. Process until you have a nice thick salsa.

7. Add salt flakes and cracked pepper to taste and set aside (the salsa can be made ahead of time and kept covered in the refrigerator; simply reheat to warm before serving).

8. To make the cashew cream, drain the soaked cashew nuts and add them to a food processor along with olive oil, lime juice, and chili sauce or tomato paste. Process on high until the nuts form a smooth cream. Taste test and add more lime juice and chili, if desired, and season with salt flakes and cracked pepper to taste. Set aside in the refrigerator.

9. Prepare the slaw by combining the shredded cabbage and grated apple in a large bowl. Make the dressing by whisking the mayonnaise with the olive oil, lime juice, and honey or agave nectar, along with salt flakes and cracked pepper to taste, until smooth.

10. Toss the dressing through the cabbage and apple and set aside, covered, in the refrigerator.

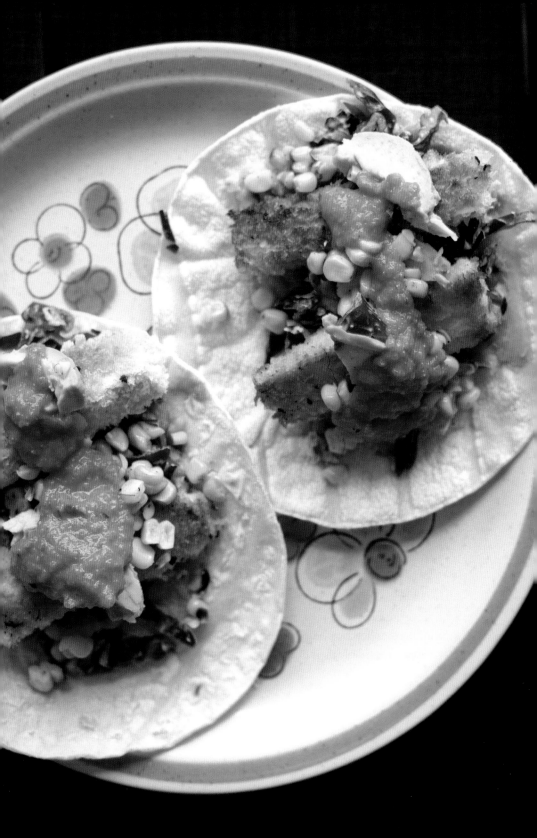

11. Place the whole ears of corn onto a lightly oiled and hot barbecue grill or stovetop grill pan. Drizzle with the olive oil and sprinkle with the spices and a good pinch each of salt flakes and cracked pepper.

12. Grill the corn on medium-high heat, turning to coat in the oil and spices until the kernels begin to reach a golden color. Remove from the pan once golden on all sides and allow the cobs to cool a little. Once cool enough to handle, run a knife down the edge of the cobs to remove the kernels. Place the grilled corn kernels into a bowl and toss with the lime and chopped cilantro. Cover and keep warm.

13. Add the chia seeds to the ¼ cup water and set aside for a few minutes until it forms a gel.

14. Slice tofu into 4-inch (10-centimeter) long strips, approximately ½ inch (1 centimeter) thick x 1 inch (2 centimeters) wide and lay in a single layer on paper towels. Top with another piece of paper towel and pat the tofu dry.

15. Combine the crumbs with the ground cumin in a shallow bowl. Fill another shallow bowl with the flour and then a third bowl with the chia gel.

16. Working with one piece of tofu at a time, finely coat with flour and then dunk in the chia gel, shaking to remove any excess before rolling in the crumbs to coat evenly. Repeat with the remaining strips of tofu, making sure your crumbs aren't too thick, or they may fall off when frying.

17. To deep-fry the tofu you need a good heavy pot with oil up to a depth of about 6 inches (15 centimeters). Heat the oil carefully over high heat until you begin to see the surface shimmer. Test the oil by adding a small piece of crumb—the oil is ready when the crumb fries instantly.

18. Working in small batches of two or three strips of breaded tofu, carefully place them in the hot oil and fry until golden on all sides. Remove with a slotted spoon and place on paper towels. Keep warm while you fry the remainder.

19. To serve the tacos, heat the tortillas until warm. Place all the ingredients, including the sliced avocado and extra wedges of lime, out on the table for everyone to assemble their own.

HOLIDAYS, PARTIES, PICNICS, AND GATHERINGS

Soy and Szechuan Pepper Tofu with Wasabi Pea Puree

PREP TIME: 45 MINUTES • SERVES: 4–6

If you're able to get your hands on fresh wasabi, by all means use it for the pea puree—simply adjust the amount to taste. Rice crumbs should be readily available in the gluten-free or health section of your supermarket or from any good natural foods store. You can substitute with panko or traditional breadcrumbs if you prefer.

PERFECT FOR NEW VEGETARIANS • SOY PROTEIN • GREAT FOR ENTERTAINING • DIFFICULTY LEVEL ***

SOY AND SZECHUAN PEPPER TOFU

1 pound (450 grams) firm tofu

juice from 1 lemon

2 teaspoons soy sauce

½ cup rice crumbs (or panko)

3 teaspoons Szechuan peppercorns, freshly ground

½ teaspoon white pepper

¼ teaspoon salt flakes

1 teaspoon cornstarch

sunflower oil, for deep-frying

WASABI PEA PUREE

2½ cups peas (fresh or frozen)

½ cup water

1–1½ teaspoons wasabi paste, to taste

1–3 tablespoons egg-free mayonnaise (optional)

ADDITIONAL INGREDIENTS

salt flakes and cracked black pepper, to taste

lemon wedges

1. Prepare the tofu by slicing the block into approximately ¼-inch (1 centimeter) deep x ¾-inch (2 centimeters) wide x 4-inch (16 centimeters) long strips and toss with the lemon juice and soy sauce in a shallow bowl.

2. Set aside while you prepare the remainder of the dish.

3. Prepare the wasabi pea puree by adding the peas and water to a frying pan. Gently simmer over low heat for 5 minutes until tender and bright green.

4. Remove from the heat, rinse under cold water, and, using a fork or stick blender, puree the peas until smooth, adding the wasabi to taste. If you would like a smoother and runnier puree you can add a little mayonnaise until you reach the desired consistency. Set aside.

5. Prepare the rice crumbs by combing well with the Szechuan pepper, white pepper, and salt flakes. Remove the tofu from the lemon juice and soy (reserving this) and pat dry with paper towels.

6. Combine the cornstarch with the reserved lemon juice and soy, whisking until smooth.

7. In a medium, deep saucepan, pour in the oil to a depth of around 6 inches (15 centimeters). Heat on high until the surface begins to shimmer.

8. Working with one piece at a time, dunk the tofu into the cornstarch mixture, shaking to remove the excess, and then roll in the rice crumbs, pressing and patting to coat the tofu evenly.

9. In small batches, deep-fry the breaded tofu for 1 minute until it is crisp and golden. Remove from the oil and drain on paper towels. Fry only a few pieces of the breaded tofu at a time to avoid overcrowding the oil.

10. Serve the tofu sprinkled with extra salt flakes, a few cracks of pepper, and wedges of lemon. Accompany with the wasabi pea puree and a crunchy side salad, like the Sprout Salad on page 133.

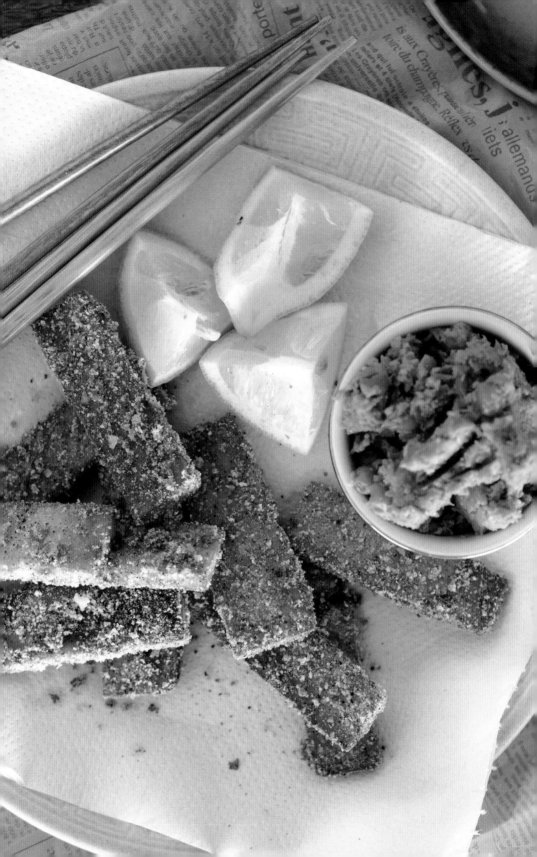

Red Lentil Sausage Rolls

PREP TIME: 80 MINUTES • SERVES: 12–18 AS AN APPETIZER
(MAKES AROUND 80 MINI SAUSAGE ROLLS)

Try serving the mini sausage rolls with Quick Tomato Relish, or use your favorite homemade or store-bought variety. For a family dinner try making larger meal-sized sausage rolls—simply increase the cooking time a little. The prepared sausage rolls are suitable to freeze, making them perfect for entertaining. Choose puff pastry labeled as suitable for vegetarians, and strict vegetarians should look for one of the vegan-friendly varieties.

PERFECT FOR NEW VEGETARIANS • LEGUME PROTEIN • GREAT FOR ENTERTAINING • SOY PROTEIN • DIFFICULTY LEVEL ***

4½ cups water

1 teaspoon curry powder

1½ cups red lentils, rinsed

½ cup pine nuts

1 red onion, quartered

2 garlic cloves, peeled

2 carrots, roughly chopped

1 tablespoons sunflower oil

½ teaspoon fresh thyme leaves

2 tablespoons mango chutney (or try tomato relish or tomato paste)

salt flakes and cracked pepper

2 pounds (1 kilogram) vegan or vegetarian-ready rolled puff pastry

½ cup nondairy milk

1–2 tablespoons poppy seeds

Quick Tomato Relish (page 80) or chutney, to serve

1. Bring the water and curry powder to a boil in a saucepan. Add the lentils, cover, and simmer gently on low for 20 minutes, until the lentils are just tender.

2. Transfer to a fine-mesh strainer and cool completely, stirring occasionally. Some of the excess liquid from the lentils should drain away, leaving a very thick consistency, once completely cooled.

3. Preheat the oven 400°F (200°C) and line two large baking trays with baking paper.

4. Meanwhile, dry roast the pine nuts over low heat in a heavy frying pan until golden. Transfer to a large bowl and set aside.

5. Place the red onion, garlic, and carrots in a food processor, and pulse on high until finely diced (alternatively, you can do this by hand).

6. In the same frying pan you dry roasted the pine nuts in, heat the sunflower oil over medium-high heat and fry the onion and carrot mixture for 3–5 minutes until soft.

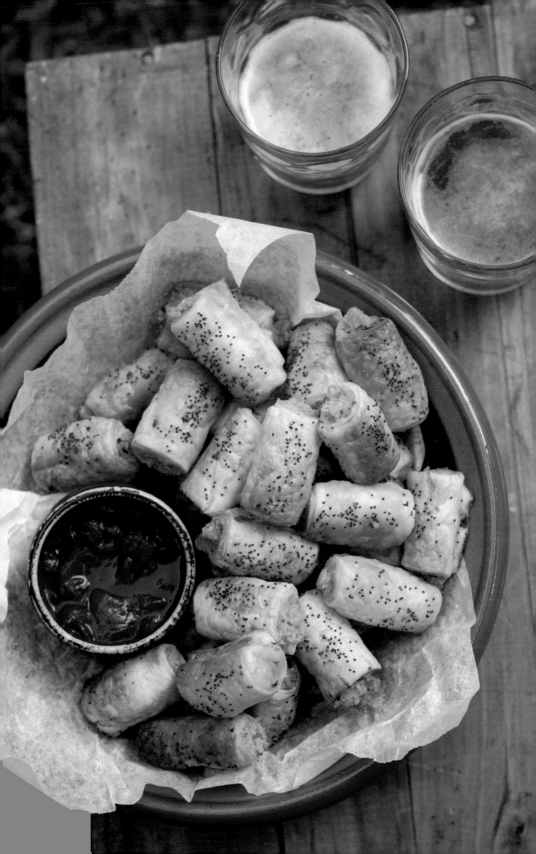

7. Add the onion and carrot mixture to the large bowl with the pine nuts. Once cool, add the thyme leaves and mango chutney (or tomato relish or tomato paste) and the cooled lentils.

8. Season with salt flakes and cracked pepper to taste and combine well.

9. Cut the sheets of puff pastry into 3½ x 2-inch (9 x 5-centimeter) strips. Working with one strip at a time, place a small teaspoon of the filling at one end and roll up, sealing over at the end with a light brush of nondairy milk. Alternatively, you can use larger strips of pastry to make meal-sized sausage rolls if you prefer. (The prepared sausage rolls can now be placed in the freezer for up to a month.)

10. Arrange the prepared sausage rolls on the baking trays. Brush each sausage roll with a little more nondairy milk and sprinkle with poppy seeds.

11. Place in the hot oven for 15 minutes until the pastry is crisp and golden. Serve hot, accompanied by tomato relish or chutney of your choice.

Trio of Pizzas

ZUCCHINI AND ASPARAGUS WITH KALE PESTO, WALNUT PASTE, AND PINE NUTS

KALE PESTO AND POTATO WITH WALNUT PASTE AND FRESH ARUGULA

SWEET POTATO AND SAGE WITH KALE PESTO AND WALNUT PASTE

PREP TIME: 40 MINUTES (PLUS 1–2 HOURS RISING TIME FOR THE DOUGH) • SERVES: 4–6

You can use store-brought pizza bases to save time, or try whipping these up with pita bread or tortillas as a quick and simple base. The Kale Pesto and Walnut Paste can be made up to 24 hours ahead. The pizza dough recipe makes three good medium-sized pizzas.

> PERFECT FOR NEW VEGETARIANS • PACKED WITH VEGGIE POWER • GREAT FOR ENTERTAINING • DIFFICULTY LEVEL **

PIZZA DOUGH

¼ ounce (7 grams) active dry yeast

1 teaspoon raw sugar

10.5 fluid ounces (300 milliliters) lukewarm water

1 pound (450 grams) bread flour or 00 flour

½ teaspoon salt flakes

2 tablespoons olive oil

ZUCCHINI AND ASPARAGUS WITH KALE PESTO, WALNUT PASTE, AND PINE NUTS

2 tablespoons Walnut Paste (page 81)

2 tablespoons tomato paste

1 small zucchini, sliced

1 bunch young asparagus, woody ends removed

2–3 tablespoons Kale Pesto (page 81)

drizzle of olive oil

1 tablespoon pine nuts

pinch of salt flakes and cracked pepper

fresh basil leaves, for garnish

KALE PESTO AND POTATO WITH WALNUT PASTE AND FRESH ARUGULA

4 tablespoons Kale Pesto (page 81)

1 small potato, thinly sliced

a few thin slices red onion

2 tablespoons red bell pepper, diced

2 tablespoons Walnut Paste (page 81)

drizzle of olive oil

salt flakes and cracked pepper

handful of fresh baby arugula

SWEET POTATO AND SAGE WITH KALE PESTO AND WALNUT PASTE

2 tablespoons Walnut Paste (page 81)

2 tablespoons Kale Pesto (page 81)

5–8 thin slices sweet potato

a few slices red onion

2–3 fresh sage leaves, torn

vegetarian feta cheese (optional)

drizzle of olive oil

salt flakes and cracked pepper, to taste

a few fresh thyme sprigs

1. To prepare the pizza dough, add the dry yeast and sugar to the lukewarm water and set aside for a few minutes until the yeast begins to react (you'll see a foam forming on the surface of the water).

2. Sift the flour and salt flakes into a large bowl, making a well in the center and adding the yeast mixture. Drizzle the olive oil around the outside of the flour.

3. Work the mixture together with your fingertips to form a mass. When the mixture has come together, turn it out onto a lightly floured surface and knead for 10 minutes until the dough is smooth and elastic.

4. Roll into a ball and place in a large bowl lightly greased with olive oil. Cover with a damp tea towel and set aside for 1–2 hours, until the dough has doubled in size.

5. Turn the dough out onto a lightly floured surface. Divide into 3 or 4 equal portions.

6. Using a lightly floured rolling pin, roll out each portion of dough at a time until thin. Transfer onto a lightly oiled and preferably preheated baking tray or pizza stone. Top with your pizza toppings.

7. While the dough is rising you can prepare the remainder of the ingredients. Setting the oven to preheat to 400°F (200°C) a good 10 or so minutes before your pizzas are ready to go in.

8. To prepare the zucchini and asparagus pizza, mix the 2 tablespoons of walnut paste with the tomato paste and smooth evenly over the prepared pizza base. Top with slices of zucchini and asparagus and then small dollops of the kale pesto. Drizzle with the olive oil, scatter with the pine nuts, and sprinkle with a little pinch of salt flakes and cracked pepper. Place in the hot oven for 10–15 minutes until the base is crisp and the toppings are golden. Remove from the oven and serve hot, drizzled with a little extra olive oil and a scatter of fresh basil leaves.

9. Make the potato pizza by spreading the prepared base with the 4 tablespoons of kale pesto. Top with slices of potato and red onion. Scatter with the bell pepper and crumble the walnut paste on top. Drizzle with a little olive oil and

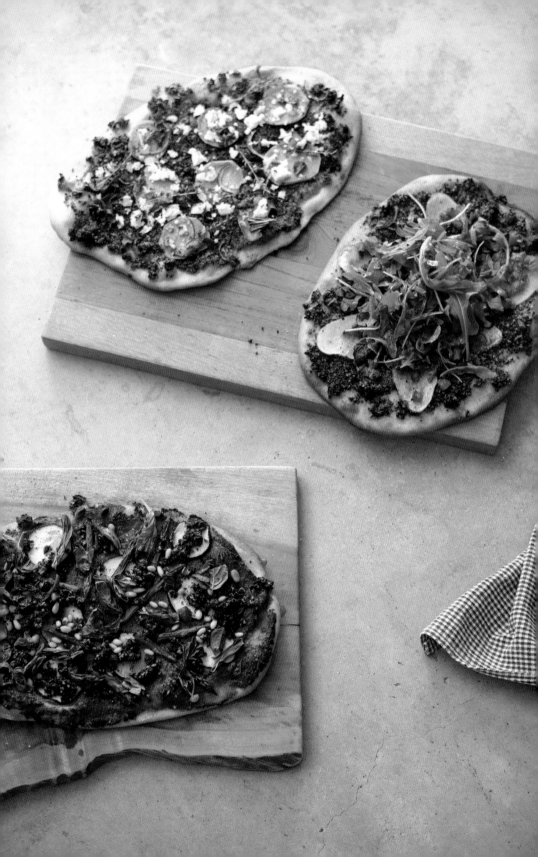

a pinch of salt flakes and cracked pepper. Place in the hot oven for 10–15 minutes, removing once the base is crisp. Serve hot piled with the fresh arugula and an extra drizzle of olive oil.

10. Prepare the sweet potato pizza by combining the walnut paste and kale pesto together before spreading over the prepared pizza base. Top with sliced sweet potato and red onion. Scatter over with the sage leaves and feta cheese, if using. Drizzle with olive oil and a pinch of salt flakes and cracked pepper. Place in the hot oven for 10–15 minutes until the base is crisp. Remove and serve hot scattered with fresh thyme and a little drizzle of olive oil.

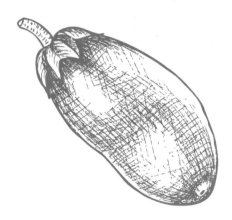

Barbecued Piri Piri Pumpkin and Tofu Skewers with Date and Walnut Couscous

PREP TIME: 40 MINUTES • SERVES: 4–6 (MAKES 12 SKEWERS)

The amount of heat in this dish will depend on the chilies you use and whether or not you seed them. If you prefer a milder piri piri, try substituting one or two red bell peppers for the chilies. You can experiment with different vegetables here. If you enjoy dairy, try swapping the tofu for cubes of vegetarian halloumi.

PERFECT FOR NEW VEGETARIANS • WHOLE-GRAIN GOODNESS • PACKED WITH VEGGIE POWER • GREAT FOR ENTERTAINING • DIFFICULTY LEVEL **

BARBECUED PIRI PIRI PUMPKIN AND TOFU SKEWERS

6 Thai red chilies

2 whole unpeeled garlic cloves

⅓ cup olive oil

1 tablespoon smoked paprika

3 tablespoons apple cider vinegar

½ teaspoon dark brown sugar

1-pound (750-gram) piece of pumpkin, peeled, seeded, and cubed

9 ounces (250 grams) firm tofu, cubed

1–2 tablespoons sunflower oil

small bunch of fresh mint and basil leaves, shredded

fresh lemon wedges, to serve

DATE AND WALNUT COUSCOUS

2 cups vegetable stock

2 cups whole wheat couscous

1 teaspoon ground cinnamon

½ cup lemon juice

3 tablespoons olive oil

10 fresh dates, roughly diced

1 cup raw walnuts, roughly chopped

1 cup loosely packed mint leaves, shredded

1. Preheat the oven to 350°F (180°C) and, if cooking the skewers on a barbecue, be sure to presoak 12 bamboo skewers now.

2. Prick the chilies with a fork and throw them into a baking tray along with the unpeeled garlic cloves. Roast in a preheated oven for 5–10 minutes until soft and golden.

3. Remove the tray from the oven and allow the chilies to cool before roughly chopping them (you can seed them now if you prefer a milder sauce), and squeeze the garlic from their skins.

4. Heat the olive oil in a frying pan over medium-low heat; add the chopped chilies, whole garlic, paprika, vinegar, and sugar. Gently simmer over low heat for about 5 minutes until the sauce has reduced and caramelized slightly.

5. Remove from the heat and allow to cool before processing in a food processor until smooth; set aside. The piri piri sauce can be prepared ahead of time and kept covered in the refrigerator.

6. Steam the cubes of pumpkin for 3–4 minutes only (until a skewer inserted easily slides through). You don't want to oversteam the pieces and turn them to mush, so watch them carefully.

7. Toss the steamed and cooled cubes of pumpkin and tofu with the prepared piri piri sauce until well coated (again, you can prepare this ahead of time and allow to marinate in the refrigerator for a few hours before cooking).

8. Thread alternating pieces of pumpkin and tofu onto the skewers and set aside.

9. To prepare the couscous, bring the 2 cups of stock to a boil in a medium saucepan. Add the couscous and stir once. Remove from the heat and set aside, covered, for around 5 minutes, until the liquid is absorbed. Using a fork, fluff the couscous to separate the grains.

10. Whisk the ground cinnamon with the lemon juice and olive oil and then toss with the dates, walnuts, mint, and prepared couscous until well combined. Set aside.

11. Heat a small amount of sunflower oil on a barbecue grill or in a stovetop grill pan. Cook the skewers in batches over a medium heat, turning until golden on all sides.

12. Remove from the heat and serve warm, scattered with the fresh herbs, lemon wedges, and the date and walnut couscous.

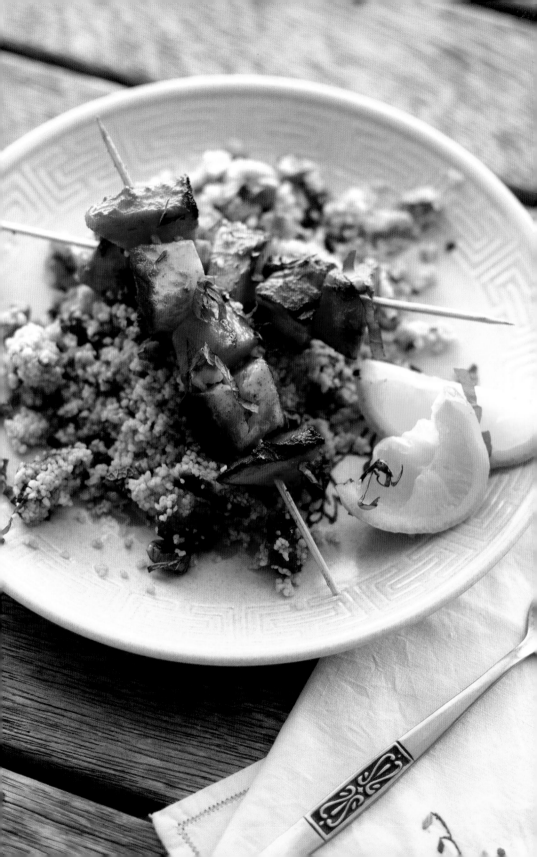

Heirloom Tomato and Onion Jam Tart with Thyme, Olive Oil, and Buckwheat Crust

PREP TIME: 55 MINUTES (PLUS 45 MINUTES OF COOKING TIME) • SERVES: 6–8

The onion jam and pastry can be made up to two days ahead. Keep the onion jam in a sealed jar or container in the refrigerator. If preparing the pastry ahead of time, do not roll it out, and cover the ball with plastic wrap. Keep in the refrigerator and remove at least 10 minutes before you are ready to use it. Look for heirloom tomatoes at your local market, but any small, sweet tomato would work well here.

> WHOLE-GRAIN GOODNESS • GREAT FOR
> ENTERTAINING • DIFFICULTY LEVEL ***

THYME, OLIVE OIL, AND BUCKWHEAT CRUST

2 cups buckwheat flour

¼ cup cornstarch

¼ teaspoon salt flakes

3 sprigs fresh thyme

1 teaspoon chia seeds

cracked pepper

¾ cup coconut oil, softened

1 tablespoon olive oil

⅓ cup chilled water (plus more, if necessary)

ONION JAM

5 yellow onions

3 tablespoons olive oil

½ teaspoon cumin seeds

¼ teaspoon salt flakes

¼ cup balsamic vinegar

2 tablespoons honey or agave nectar

ADDITIONAL INGREDIENTS

20 ounces (600 grams) mixed variety small heirloom tomatoes

1 tablespoon olive oil

pinch of salt flakes and cracked pepper

fresh basil leaves, to serve

1. To make the pastry, sift the flours into a large bowl add the salt flakes, leaves from the thyme sprigs, chia seeds, and cracked pepper to taste. Combine well.

2. Dollop the coconut oil and drizzle the olive oil evenly over the flour. Using a knife, cut the oil into the flour until it clumps into pea-sized balls.

3. Slowly drip the chilled water into the flour mixture, working with your hands after each tablespoon of water added, until the pastry just begins to hold together (you may need more or less than the ⅓ cup of water). Roll the pastry into a ball.

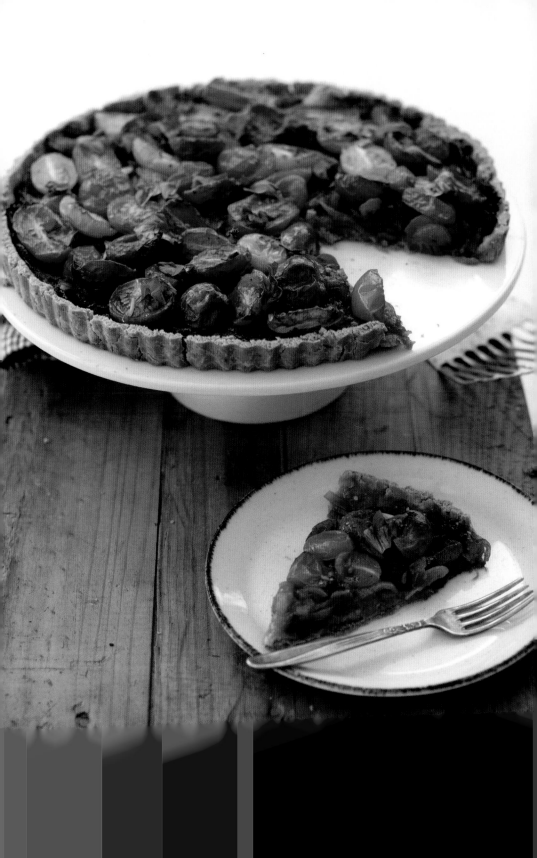

4. Lightly dust a clean work surface and rolling pin with a little extra buckwheat flour. Lightly dust the dough just enough to stop everything from sticking together and then carefully roll out your pastry, pinching any tears back together. Work gently with the pastry until you have an approximately 14-inch (35-centimeter) diameter circle.

5. Laying the pastry over your rolling pin, carefully transfer to a 10¾-inch (27-centimeter) tart pan with a removable bottom. Press the pastry into the tart pan, pinching and patting any tears back together. Trim the edges. Set the prepared pastry in the refrigerator while you make the onion jam.

6. Peel, halve, and thinly slice the onions. Heat the oil over a low heat in a heavy pan with a lid. Add the cumin seeds and toss for just a minute. Add the onions and salt, and over low heat, "sweat" the onions with the lid on, tossing occasionally for 10 minutes, until soft.

7. Continue to cook the onions over low heat, stirring frequently with the lid off, for 15 minutes. The onions will start to golden and become very soft.

8. Increase the heat to medium and add the balsamic vinegar and honey or agave nectar, stirring to combine well. Turn down the heat to low again and cook gently for 30–35 minutes, stirring occasionally, until you have a syrupy jam. Remove from the heat and allow to cool.

9. While the onion jam is cooking, preheat the oven to 325°F (170°C) and slice the tomatoes in half.

10. Toss the sliced tomatoes with the olive oil and a good pinch each of salt flakes and cracked pepper. Set aside.

11. Once the onion jam is ready, remove the prepared crust from the refrigerator. Fill the tart crust with the cooled onion jam and then top with the sliced tomatoes in a single layer to fill the entire tart.

12. Place in the preheated oven for 40–45 minutes until the tomatoes are blistered and golden. Remove from the oven and cool slightly before serving, scattered with torn basil leaves.

13. Makes a lovely meal served with a simple salad of dressed greens.

Crispy Fried Polenta with Baby Kale and Sundried Tomatoes

PREP TIME: 45 MINUTES (PLUS 1 HOUR REFRIGERATION) • SERVES: 4–6

Both the dressing and the polenta can be prepared ahead of time and kept covered in the refrigerator, making the salad perfect for entertaining or an easy "prep ahead" midweek meal.

WHOLE-GRAIN GOODNESS • PACKED WITH VEGGIE POWER
• GREAT FOR ENTERTAINING • DIFFICULTY LEVEL **

1 quart (1 liter) vegetable stock

1 cup polenta (coarse cornmeal)

½ cup extra cornmeal

1–2 tablespoons sunflower oil

12 ounces (350 grams) sundried tomatoes, roughly chopped

4 ounces (120 grams) baby kale

2½ ounces (75 grams) baby spinach

1 avocado, sliced and drizzled with lemon juice

¼ cup sunflower seeds

FOR THE DRESSING

3 tablespoons egg-free mayonnaise

3 tablespoons olive oil

1 tablespoons apple cider vinegar

½–1 teaspoon grated horseradish (or horseradish cream), to taste

½ teaspoon honey or agave nectar

salt flakes and cracked pepper, to taste

1. To prepare the polenta, bring the stock to boil in a large saucepan. Once boiling, add the polenta in a steady stream, whisking continually until well combined.

2. Reduce the heat to very low and continue to cook for 10–15 minutes, stirring with a wooden spoon until thick and smooth. The polenta is cooked when the grains are soft and tender.

3. Pour the hot polenta into a 10½-pint or 6-liter capacity lightly greased baking dish. Smooth over the top and refrigerate for about an hour until set.

4. To make the dressing, whisk all the ingredients together until combined. Set aside.

5. Once the polenta is set, turn it out of the dish and cut into pieces around 2 x ¼-inch (5 x 1-centimeter) thick. Dust each piece with the extra cornmeal.

6. Heat 1 tablespoon of the sunflower oil in a heavy frying pan over medium heat. Working in small batches, fry the squares of prepared polenta over

medium-high heat for a few minutes until golden. Turn each piece and continue to fry until golden on both sides. Transfer to paper towels and fry the remaining pieces, adding more oil to the pan if needed.

7. Cut each square of fried polenta diagonally to make triangles.

8. Gently toss the prepared fried polenta and sundried tomatoes together with the baby kale, baby spinach, sliced avocado, and sunflower seeds in a large bowl.

9. Just before serving, pile the salad onto a serving plate and drizzle with the dressing.

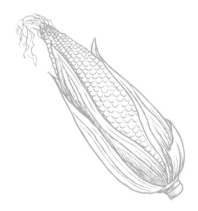

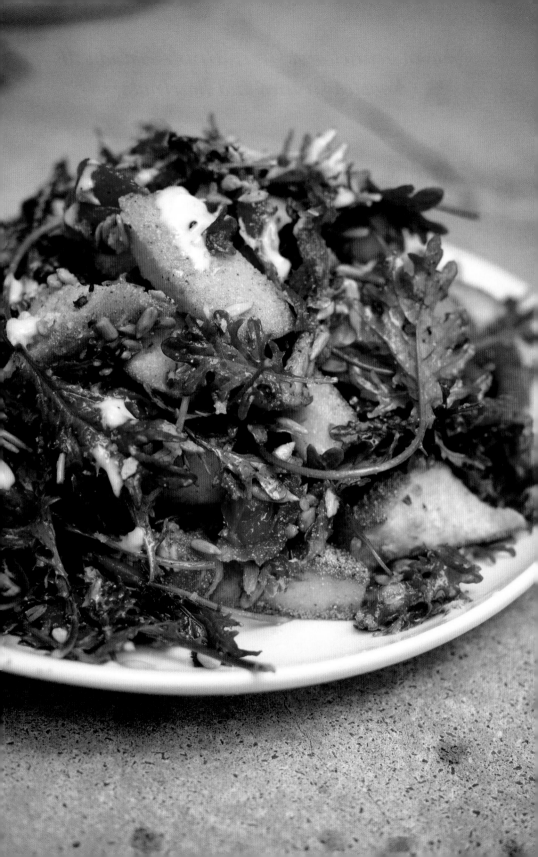

Shaved Fennel and Green Apple Salad with Roasted Grapes and Hazelnuts

PREP TIME: 35 MINUTES • SERVES: 4 AS A SIDE

This salad makes a lovely addition to traditional holiday fare and is also a great accompaniment to the Red Lentil Sausage Rolls (page 164).

PACKED WITH VEGGIE POWER • GREAT FOR ENTERTAINING • DIFFICULTY LEVEL *

7 ounces (200 grams) red seedless grapes

3½ ounces (100 grams) hazelnuts

1 tablespoon walnut oil

3 teaspoons fresh thyme leaves, divided

2 green apples

juice from ½ lemon

1 medium fennel bulb

ORANGE AND WALNUT OIL DRESSING

2 tablespoons fresh orange juice

3 tablespoons walnut oil

½ teaspoon honey or agave nectar

1 teaspoon apple cider vinegar

salt flakes and cracked pepper, to taste

1. Preheat the oven to 350°F (180°C).

2. Throw the grapes and hazelnuts into a baking tray. Drizzle with the walnut oil and 2 teaspoons of the thyme leaves. Toss to coat well and the pop in the preheated oven for 10–15 minutes, until the grapes just begin to blister. Remove from the oven and allow to cool.

3. Meanwhile core, halve, and thinly slice the apples, tossing in lemon juice before transferring to a large bowl. Remove the outer parts of the fennel and then thinly slice the bulb, discarding the leafy tops. Add the fennel to the sliced apple.

4. Reserving a few of the hazelnuts for garnish, add the cooled grapes and nuts to the fennel and apple and gently toss to combine.

5. To make the dressing, whisk all the ingredients together in a small bowl.

6. Dress the salad just before serving. Arrange the dressed salad on a platter and top with remaining thyme leaves and reserved nuts.

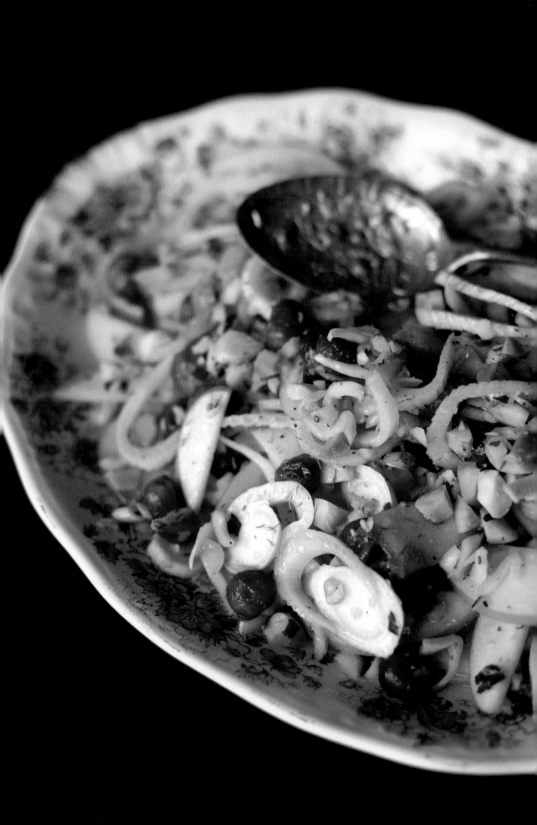

Spicy Lentil Tart with Pomegranate and Mint

PREP TIME: 40 MINUTES • SERVES: 4

Be sure to check the ingredients on ready-rolled puff pastry, as not all will be vegetarian/vegan. For a complete meal, serve with the Date and Walnut Couscous (page 171) and a side of lightly dressed leafy greens.

PERFECT FOR NEW VEGETARIANS • LEGUME PROTEIN • GREAT FOR ENTERTAINING • DIFFICULTY LEVEL **

3 cups vegetable stock

2 bay leaves

½ cinnamon stick

1 cup brown lentils, rinsed

1 teaspoon black peppercorns

½ teaspoon salt flakes

1 teaspoon cumin seeds

1 teaspoon paprika

½ teaspoon coriander seeds

1 tablespoon pomegranate molasses or blackstrap molasses

1 tablespoon warm water

9-inch (24-centimeter) squared sheet of pre-made vegetarian puff pastry

¼ cup soy milk

1 tablespoon sunflower oil

1 tablespoon olive oil

½ red onion, finely diced

½ cup pine nuts

1 cup flat-leaf parsley, roughly chopped

1 cup fresh mint, roughly chopped

1 red chili, seeded and diced (optional)

1 teaspoon sumac

seeds from ½ pomegranate

TO SERVE

½ cup tahini

1 tablespoon olive oil

juice from 1 lemon

1 tablespoon water

1 lemon, cut into wedges

1. Preheat the oven to 350°F (180°C).

2. Bring the stock, bay leaves, and cinnamon stick to a boil in a large pot. Add the lentils and turn down the heat. Simmer gently, covered, for 15–20 minutes, stirring occasionally until the lentils are tender and the liquid has absorbed. Remove the bay leaves and cinnamon stick, straining off any excess liquid, and set aside.

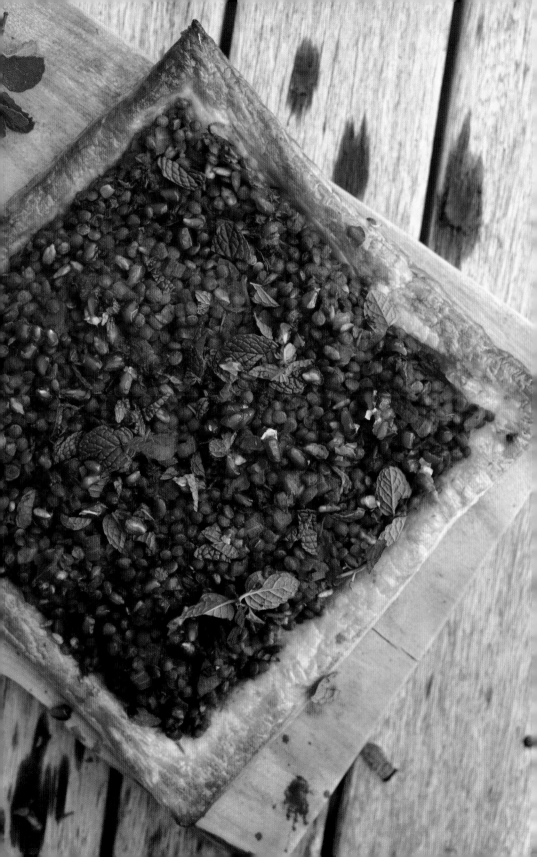

3. Heat a small saucepan over low heat. Add the pine nuts and dry roast in a single layer, tossing frequently for a few minutes until golden. Remove from the heat and set aside.

4. Grind the black peppercorns, salt flakes, cumin seeds, paprika, and coriander seeds together in a mortar and pestle to form a fine spice powder.

5. Combine the pomegranate molasses with 1 tablespoon of warm water until smooth, and set aside.

6. Lay the puff pastry sheet on a lightly greased baking tray lined with baking paper. Carefully score a 1-inch (3-centimeter) border around the outside of the pastry sheet with a knife. Using a pastry brush, brush the pastry border with a little soy milk.

7. Place the prepared pastry sheet in the preheated oven and bake for 10 minutes, until the pastry just begins to puff and golden. Remove from the oven and set aside.

8. Meanwhile, heat the sunflower and olive oil in a heavy frying pan and fry the onion over medium heat for a few minutes until soft. Add the prepared spice powder and continue to cook for a few minutes until fragrant. Add the prepared lentils and toss well to combine.

9. Add the pomegranate molasses and water mixture, plus the pine nuts, and continue to cook for another 4–5 minutes, until the lentils just begin to brown and stick to the bottom of the pan. Remove from the heat, add the fresh herbs, reserving half the mint, plus the diced red chili, if using, and stir though.

10. Spoon the lentil mixture onto the prepared puff pastry sheet, leaving the border around the edge. Sprinkle with the sumac and return to the oven for 15 minutes until pastry is golden.

11. Meanwhile, whisk the tahini paste with the olive oil, lemon juice, and water until smooth, adding more water if needed to reach a smooth consistency.

12. Remove the tart from the oven. Serve sprinkled with pomegranate seeds and reserved mint. Accompany with the tahini dressing and wedges of fresh lemon.

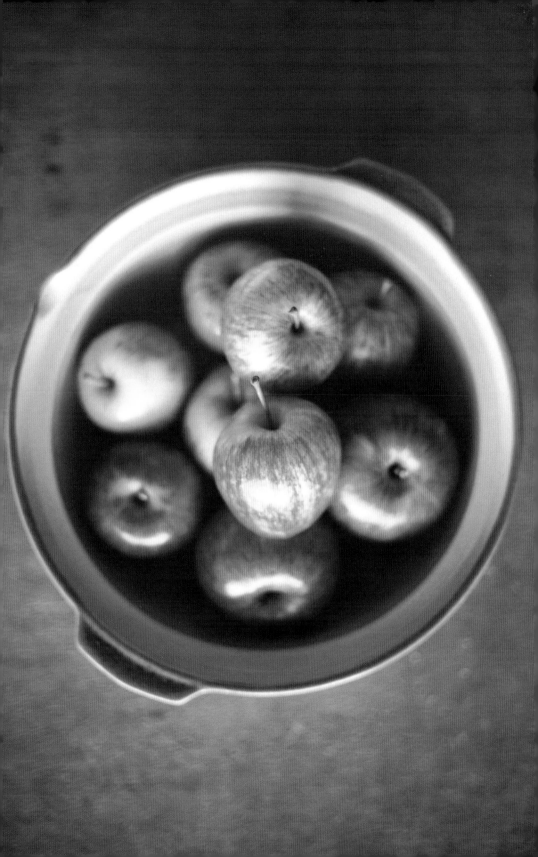

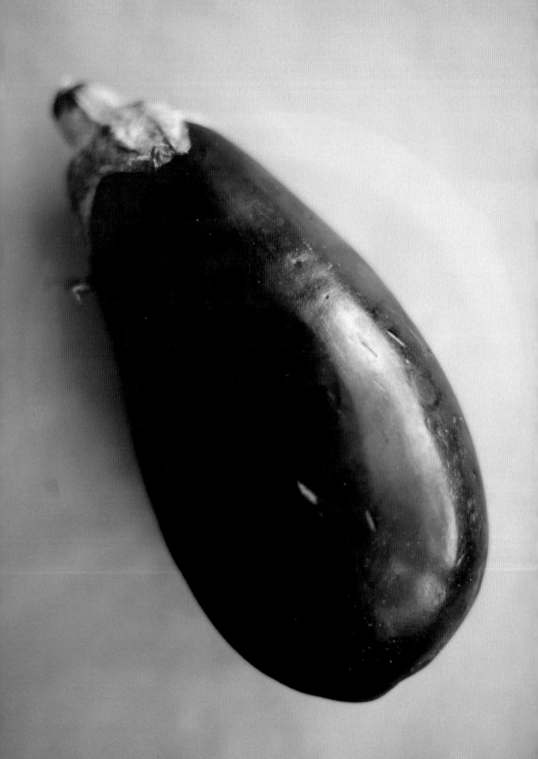

GLOSSARY

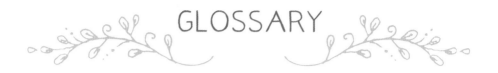

Agave Nectar

Agave nectar, or more accurately agave syrup, is a sweetener made from the agave plant. A little sweeter and thinner than honey, it makes a good substitute for those looking to avoid all animal products. You'll find agave nectar in heath food and natural foods stores; or, ask for it at your supermarket.

Amaranth Flour

Nutrient-rich and boasting the highest protein level of any grain, amaranth is also a good source of calcium, iron, magnesium, and fiber. Best used in combination with other flours. Look for amaranth flour at your health food or natural foods store.

Arborio Rice

Also called risotto rice, arborio rice is a short, fat variety of rice perfect for use in risotto, as it holds together even after absorbing a large amount of liquid. Look for arborio rice with other rice varieties at your supermarket.

Arugula

Arugula is a leafy salad green with a mustard/peppery taste perfect for salads and vegetable dishes. The younger leaves have a milder flavor and can often be found in salad combinations with baby spinach and other salad greens. Available as bunches or loose leaves at your local fruit and vegetable market or supermarket. Best used when very fresh. Look for arugula with bright green leaves and store covered in the refrigerator for only a few days.

Baby Spinach

Simply the young or immature leaves of the spinach plant, baby spinach is delicate, tender, and has a sweeter flavor than mature spinach. It's perfect for use in salads, wraps, and sandwiches. Look for loose leaves of baby spinach available at your fruit and vegetable market or supermarket. Choose fresh, healthy, and dark green leaves. Store covered in your refrigerator and use within a few days.

Beets

Beets are a delicious and super-nutritious root vegetable full of beautiful flavor and rich color. Both the root and leaves, which are similar to spinach, can be eaten and provide a wealth of antioxidants, vitamins, and minerals. Look for smaller beets with their whiskers and dark healthy leaves intact. A delicious vegetable grated in fresh salads, roasted, steamed, or served in soups.

Blackstrap Molasses

A by-product of the sugar-refining process, blackstrap molasses is thick, bittersweet syrup perfect in both savory and sweet dishes. Nutrient dense, it provides a wealth of essential minerals, including a good dose of iron and calcium. Look for it alongside honey and syrups on the supermarket shelf or in any good health food store.

Bok Choy

Bok choy is one of the many varieties of leafy Chinese vegetables. With crisp pale stems and mild tasting green leaves, bok choy, also known as pak choy or pak choi, is very similar to baby bok choy. You'll find bok choy at Asian food stores that sell fresh fruit and vegetables, good fruit and vegetables markets, and supermarkets. Choose bunches with bright green and healthy leaves with firm stems. Keep covered in your refrigerator and use within a few days.

Broccolini

Broccolini is a hybrid between broccoli and Chinese kale. Similar to broccoli but with smaller florets and longer stalks, it is sweeter, with a delicate, almost peppery taste. Look for bunches of broccolini at your local farmer's market or supermarket. Choose those bright green in color and with firm stems. Substitute with broccoli if broccolini is unavailable.

Buckwheat Flour

Despite its deceptive name, buckwheat is actually a seed, making buckwheat flour ideal for those sensitive to gluten—plus, it is a source of essential minerals and fiber. Buckwheat flour has a slight gray tinge and lovely, subtle earthy flavor. Find it at any good natural foods store, or try searching for buckwheat flour in your supermarket along with other gluten-free items.

Buckwheat Groats (Raw)

Raw buckwheat groats are small, triangular kernels of the buckwheat plant. They are pale brown to green in color and available from any good natural foods store or supermarket. Versatile and easy to prepare, buckwheat groats store well sealed in a jars or containers in your pantry.

Cacao (Raw Cacao Powder/Cacao Nibs)

Not to be confused with processed cocoa or cocoa powder, raw cacao is not roasted, relatively unprocessed, and contains no sugar or other added ingredients. Raw cacao is available as both powder and nibs from your local health food or natural foods store and increasingly in supermarkets. Rich in antioxidants, raw cacao is also a source of iron, zinc, folate, and magnesium. A good ingredient used sparingly in things like smoothies, raw desserts, bars, and cookies.

Chia Seeds

These tiny black or white seeds are available at your local health food and natural foods store or in the health aisle of your supermarket. They are gluten-free and a great source of vegetarian fiber, omega-3, protein, antioxidants, calcium, iron, and potassium. Super-versatile, chia seeds can be added to your breakfast granola or oatmeal and thrown into smoothies, juices, raw desserts, bars, and cookies. Or use them to make a gel for replacing eggs in baking. As a guide, combine 1 teaspoon of chia seeds with ¼ cup of filtered water. Set aside for around 10 minutes until the chia seeds and water have formed a gooey gel. This amount of chia gel is equal to approximately one egg. Simply increase the amounts for each egg you wish to replace.

Chickpeas (Garbanzo Beans)

A versatile and super-healthy legume, chickpeas (garbanzo beans) are available as both dried or canned. Dried beans can take 1–1½ hours to cook but do have better flavor and texture than their canned counterpart. Canned beans make a great ready and quick standby— simply rinse well before use. Look for chickpeas at your natural foods store or supermarket.

Coconut Oil (Virgin)

Coconut oil is oil extracted from the meat of mature coconuts. Virgin coconut oil, sometimes labeled as raw or cold-pressed, is unrefined and should have a mild coconut flavor and scent. Coconut oil should stay soft when stored above 77°F (25°C) and will solidify into butter if stored below this or kept in the refrigerator. You'll find coconut oil at any good heath food or natural foods store. Or, ask for it at your supermarket. Virgin coconut oil should keep well stored in your pantry. In cold climates, if your coconut oil solidifies, simply place the jar in a bowl filled with hot water until it softens enough for use.

Coconut Water

Coconut water is the clear liquid found inside young coconuts, unlike coconut milk, which is made from the coconut meat. Look for pure coconut water that contains no additives, preservatives, or sweeteners, and the fresher the better. Available in heath food and natural foods stores or ask for it at your supermarket.

Coconut Yogurt

Coconut yogurt is yogurt made from coconut milk instead of dairy milk. Made in the same fashion using a starter of probiotic cultures, it offers a delicious alternative to traditional yogurt. Look for it in health food and natural foods stores. It can be a little expensive, so consider the fun option of making your own at home.

Couscous

Made from durum wheat (like most traditional pasta), couscous is a quick-to-prepare and versatile ingredient—excellent served with fresh or roasted vegetables. Typically available with other pasta products on supermarket shelves, look for whole wheat couscous for optimal nutritional value.

Curry Leaves

Curry leaves are the slightly spicy leaves of the curry plant and unrelated to curry powder. Available as both fresh and dried, the fresh are far superior in flavor and aroma. Look for fresh curry leaves at ethnic food stores or your local fruit and vegetable market. Fresh leaves can be stored in the freezer for up to three months. If you can't find fresh, look for dried curry leaves with the spices in your supermarket; simply double the quantity in recipes.

Edamame

Edamame are young soybeans usually purchased and cooked still in their pods. A great source of vegetable protein, they make a nutritious and tasty addition to a vegetarian diet. Look for them, typically available frozen, at your Asian food store, or ask for them at your supermarket.

Egg-Free Mayonnaise

There are many different varieties of egg-free mayonnaise readily available from your local natural foods store or supermarket. Some are soy-based while others are made using sunflower or other oils. It is easy to make your own at home; simply jump online to find a few recipes to test out. Those who aren't strict vegetarian can substitute traditional mayonnaise for the egg-free in all the recipes in this book.

Eggplant

There are a few main types of eggplant—all are versatile and full of rich, smoky flavor and silky texture. Look for the large, pendulum-shaped common eggplant or the slender and smaller finger or Japanese eggplant. Choose those with firm, bright, and shiny skins and keep stored in the crisper of your refrigerator for only a few days at the most. Excellent roasted, grilled, fried, or stewed.

Fennel

With a distinct anise flavor, fennel is a beautiful bulb vegetable, perfect for roasting or shaved in fresh salads. Look for small tender bulbs with healthy green leaves. Store for only a few days in the crisper of your fridge.

Flaxseeds (Linseeds)

An excellent source of omega-3 fatty acids, flaxseeds are an important ingredient to include in a healthy vegetarian diet. The raw seeds are small and typically brown or reddish in color. Great for use in cookies, breads, and homemade granola or sprinkled on salads and vegetable dishes. Look for flaxseeds at your local natural foods store or supermarket. The whole seeds will keep well, stored in a sealed jar or container in your pantry.

Harissa

Harissa is a hot and spicy paste made from roasted chilies, garlic, and spices—a fiery ingredient perfect for use in sauces and marinades. You'll find the paste available at ethnic food stores; or, try making your own—jump online to find recipes.

Hemp Seeds

While relatively new to the modern Western diet, hemp seeds have been consumed as a food throughout the world for hundreds of years. They are a balanced and easily digestible source of high-quality protein and important omega-3 and omega-6 fatty acids, are rich in antioxidants, and provide fiber, calcium, magnesium, iron, zinc, B vitamins, and vitamin E. With a slightly nutty taste, the seeds can be added to nearly any meal you can think of. Try some in smoothies and juices, sprinkled on top of your breakfast, or added to baked goods and salads. Available as a food in most countries; check your local natural foods or health foods store to see if they have hemp seeds or other hemp seed products such as hemp milk and hemp oil available.

Kale

A super-healthy and nutrient-dense leafy vegetable related to broccoli and cabbage, kale looks similar to chard. There are a few different varieties, with the curly leafed being the most widely available. Look for kale in your local supermarket or local fruit and vegetable market. Chose those with healthy, robust leaves and use within a few days of purchasing.

Lentils

Lentils are quick and easy to prepare, provide a good source of lean vegetarian protein and iron, and are a great source of fiber. Available dried as red, green, brown, and puy (French) lentils from all good natural foods stores and most supermarkets. You can also find lentils as a canned product. Although these tend to be poorer in terms of flavor and texture, they can make a super-quick standby when you don't have time to cook. Dried lentils will store for long periods in a sealed jar or container in your pantry. Always wash your lentils before use. As a guide to preparing dried lentils, bring 3 cups of water to a boil for every 1 cup of lentils. Add the lentils to the boiling water and gently simmer, covered, for 25–35 minutes, until the lentils are tender.

Miso Paste

A traditional Japanese condiment made from slowly fermented soybeans, rice, or barley. Most commonly used in soup, the salty and deliciously unique flavor of miso also works well in dressings, sauces, and marinades. Look for the lighter flavored "white" miso or the full-flavored dark or red miso at your local Asian food store or in the Asian foods aisle of your supermarket.

Mustard Seeds

Available as white, black, brown, or yellow, and as whole seeds or powder, mustard seeds are aromatic and slightly nutty. They are often fried in oil to lend their flavor to curries or used in dressings and sauces. Look for whole mustard seeds along with the spices and peppercorns in your supermarket.

Nutritional Yeast (Savory Nutritional Flakes)

With a nutty, some say cheesy, flavor, nutritional yeast is deactivated yeast available as flakes or powder from your health food or natural foods store. This versatile ingredient is great for adding both flavor and nutrition to your vegetarian meals. Good-quality nutritional yeast should contain B12 and provide a source of protein, B vitamins, selenium, and zinc.

Palm Sugar

Made from the sap of various palm trees, palm sugar is popular in Southeast Asian cuisine. You'll find palm sugar available as solid "cakes" at your local Asian food store or in the Asian food aisle of your supermarket. Brown sugar can be substituted in most recipes.

Panko

Panko or panko crumbs are Japanese breadcrumbs. Although made from whole wheat like your typical breadcrumbs, panko are lighter, with a delicate flaky texture. Look for panko at Asian food stores or in the Asian aisle at your supermarket. Perfect for a crispy coating on deep-fried foods; or, try them anywhere you would use typical breadcrumbs for a lighter and crisper result.

Patty Pan Squash

Patty pan squash are small, round, mild-tasting summer squash with scalloped edges. Available in yellow and green varieties, you should find them when in season at your local fruit and vegetable market or supermarket.

Peanut Butter (Raw)

Raw peanut butter is preferable over many processed peanut butters, in that it has no added salt or sugar. Look for raw peanut butter made from 100 percent peanuts at your local heath food or natural foods store, or try making your own—it's fun and super easy.

Pine Nuts

The edible seeds of pine trees, these slightly sweet and buttery flavored nuts are popular in both savory and sweet dishes. Beautiful when lightly toasted, you can find the raw nuts alongside other nuts and seeds in the supermarket aisle or at your natural foods store.

Polenta (Coarse Cornmeal)

Confusingly, polenta is both a term for a dish and the ingredient used to make it. Made from ground sweet corn, polenta is also often labeled as cornmeal or grits. When making polenta, choose a coarse cornmeal or one labeled as polenta. Typically yellow in color, raw polenta has a coarse, grainy texture and will store well in a sealed jar or container in your pantry. Look for polenta or coarse cornmeal with the pasta in your supermarket or natural foods store.

Pomegranate

A beautiful and antioxidant-rich fruit, pomegranates have a thick outer skin and bright jewel-like seeds inside. The juicy seeds are full of sweet/tart flavor, making them perfect for use in both savory and sweet dishes. Look for pomegranates at your local fruit and vegetable market, ethnic food store, or supermarket. Choose heavy fruit with firm skin and store in a cool place for up to two weeks.

Pumpkin Seeds (Pepitas)

A good source of zinc and iron, these nutty-tasting seeds are green in color and make an excellent and versatile addition to your vegetarian diet. Add them to nearly any kind of dish—from roasted vegetables to salads, pasta, and rice dishes, and sweet things like granola, cakes, cookies, and smoothies. You'll find pumpkin seeds with other seeds at your natural foods store or supermarket. They'll keep well stored in a sealed jar or container in your pantry.

Quinoa

Quinoa, pronounced KEEN-wah, is nutrient-rich seed more commonly stored, prepared, and eaten like a grain and as such is grouped with grains and cereals in this book. Quinoa is typically regarded as a vegetarian source of complete protein, and its distinct texture and nutty flavor makes a super-nutritious and tasty addition to many vegetarian meals. Look for white and red quinoa, now readily available in the health aisle of your supermarket or at any good natural foods store.

Quinoa Flakes

Quinoa flakes are made in the same fashion as rolled oats—by steaming and rolling the whole kernel. As such, they are similar to rolled oats and can be cooked and eaten in the same way. Quinoa flakes make a great gluten-free substitute to rolled oats in baking and at breakfast time. Look for quinoa flakes at your natural foods store or with gluten-free items at your supermarket.

Rolled Oats

Rolled oats are steamed and pressed whole oat grains. They differ from steel-cut oats in both texture and cooking time. Quick oats are also steamed and rolled, but are cut finer, so you lose some texture in baking. Look for rolled oats, sometimes called traditional or old-fashioned oats, at your natural foods store or supermarket.

Rolled Rye

Just as rolled oats, rolled rye is the steamed and pressed whole rye grain. High in fiber, keep this tasty ingredient on hand for use in homemade granola, cookies, cakes, and bread. Ask for it at your local natural foods store or substitute with rolled oats if unavailable.

Shiitake Mushrooms

Shiitake mushrooms have a "meaty" texture and full flavor, prefect for vegetarian cooking. Look for fresh sliced or whole shiitake at your local fruit and vegetable market, Asian food store, or Asian aisle of your supermarket. Dried shiitake mushrooms are wonderful for adding rich flavor to soups and broths.

Shoots and Sprouts

Easy to grow at home, you'll also find a large variety of fresh shoots and sprouts available in fruit and vegetable stores and supermarkets. An incredibly nutritious raw food, excellent for adding flavor, texture, and goodness to salads, sandwiches, and juices. Look for snow pea and bamboo shoots, bean sprouts, alfalfa sprouts, and handy combinations of mixed sprouts that often contain things like radish, mustard greens, arugula, broccoli, and more. Legume sprouts are large and crunchy and make a lovely addition to salads and sandwiches—look for lentil, mung bean, chickpea, or a combination. Keep shoots and sprouts in your refrigerator and use within a few days.

Soba Noodles

Soba noodles are a traditional Japanese noodle made from buckwheat or a combination of buckwheat and durum wheat. Versatile, tasty, and super quick to prepare, soba noodles are a great ingredient to have on hand. You'll find soba noodles at your Asian food store or in the Asian food aisle of your supermarket.

Spelt Flour

Related to wheat, spelt is a cereal grain of ancient origin. It has a nutty flavor and is slightly sweeter than typical wheat flour with a little more protein, too. You can use spelt flour as you would traditional all-purpose flour in most recipes, and it's a great way to introduce a different grain into your diet. Look for spelt flour along with the other flours in your supermarket or at any good natural foods store.

Spelt Pasta

Spelt pasta is pasta made from spelt, rather than durum wheat, the ingredient in most common pastas. It has a slightly nutty flavor and can be stored and used just as typical pasta. Look for spelt pasta in your supermarket or at your local health foods store.

Spirulina

Spirulina is an incredibly nutrient-dense algae packed with vegetable protein and a host of essential vitamins and minerals. It's available as a powder or in tablet form from your local heath food or natural foods store. It can be an expensive product, but you only need to use a little at a time—make sure you follow the recommended dosage on the packet. Spirulina will not store for long periods. After opening, use within three months and keep it stored, well sealed, in a cool dark place.

Star Anise (Star Aniseed)

Popular in Chinese and Vietnamese cooking, star anise is a dried, star-shaped fruit with a lovely aniseed or licorice flavor. Available whole or in powdered form from supermarkets and Asian food stores.

Sumac

Sumac, pronounced SOO-mak, is a spice powder of dried berries with a beautiful tangy, almost citrus flavor. Look for powdered or whole sumac in the spice section of your supermarket or at ethnic food stores.

Sunflower Seeds

Packing an impressive nutrient profile, sunflower seeds are healthy, tasty, and super versatile. The shelled pale gray seeds of the sunflower plant, they have a subtle nutty flavor and tender texture. Perfect for snacking and adding to almost anything you can think of. Look for raw sunflower seeds at your local natural foods store or supermarket. Whole seeds will keep well sealed in a jar or container in your pantry.

Szechuan Pepper

Not actually a peppercorn, but a dried berry, Szechuan pepper is popular in Asian cuisine. Aromatic rather than hot, whole or ground Szechuan pepper is available in the spice aisle of your supermarket or at your local Asian food store.

Tahini

Tahini is a smooth paste made from ground sesame seeds and is available as both hulled and unhulled tahini. The unhulled variety is richer in nutrients, darker in appearance, and has a more distinct flavor. With all the nutritional benefits of sesame seeds, including being a great dairy-free source of calcium, tahini is a versatile and delicious ingredient. Look for it at health food and natural foods stores or in the health aisle of your supermarket. Keep it stored in the pantry, not the refrigerator, as this will cause it to separate—the high oil content will keep it from going rancid.

Tamari

A rich, salty sauce made from fermented soybeans, it differs from soy sauce in that most tamari is made using little or no wheat. If often has a smoother and less salty taste than typical soy sauce—perfect for seasoning and use in sauces and marinades. Look for tamari at Asian food stores or in your supermarket, shelved with soy sauce or gluten-free items.

Tempeh

Tempeh is a fermented soy product with a firmer texture and more distinct flavor than tofu. Available in blocks in a variety of forms, often as a ready-to-eat or pre-cooked product, tempeh can also be found "flavored" with soy sauce or marinades. Look for tempeh at your local natural foods, health food, or Asian food store.

Tofu (Bean Curd)

Tofu is made from pressed soy milk curds and comes in a variety of forms. Most commonly used are silken tofu and firm tofu. Both come packaged in water and have mute flavor. Silken tofu is excellent for use in sauces, soups, and even desserts. Firm tofu can be cubed or crumbled and served baked, grilled, scrambled, or deep-fried. Or look for handy ready-to-eat marinated tofu for quick additions to noodle dishes, salads, and sandwiches. You'll find lots of tofu varieties in the cold section of your local supermarket, Asian, or natural foods store. Keep fresh tofu in the refrigerator. It's best used on the day of opening.

Turkish Apricots

Turkish apricots are usually plump, with a rich and sweeter flavor than other dried apricots. Typically dried whole, these apricots are best when preservative/sulphate free. Look for Turkish apricots at your natural foods store or supermarket.

Turmeric (Fresh)

Turmeric is a member of the ginger family and very similar in appearance to fresh ginger. Orange/brown on the outside and vibrant orange on the inside, this good-for-you ingredient is perfect for adding fresh flavor and goodness to soups, smoothies, and hot drinks. Look for it at your local Asian food store or fruit and vegetable market, or ask for it at your supermarket. Choose firm and healthy-looking pieces and grate or pound the root before use. Take care though, as the rich color of fresh turmeric can stain nearly anything it touches—countertops, hands, clothes, and porous kitchenware.

RECIPE INDEX

Please note that photographs are not indexed.

INDEX

ACKNOWLEDGMENTS

I'd love to thank all the people in my life, especially my Mum, for always taking the time to create, share, and enjoy delicious food together—to all my family and friends, thank you for your unwavering support. To each and every follower of *Veggie num num*, for all your support, comments, feedback, and love, I am so very grateful and eternally thankful. To my husband and my daughter, thank you for inspiring me each day to create wholesome veggie food to feed our bellies and keep us healthy and happy. To the team at Ulysses Press, thank you for everything. And to each one of you who've read this book, I thank you and hope you've found within its pages a little inspiration to become the healthy and happy vegetarian you hope to be.

ABOUT THE AUTHOR

Trudy Slabosz is the creator of the popular vegetarian blog *Veggie num num*. A vegetarian for more than 15 years, she has a passion for healthy vegetarian food and creating veggie meals that everyone can enjoy. Vegetarianism has had a profoundly positive effect on her life; her goal is to share just how easy, healthy, and delicious being a vegetarian can be. She lives and cooks in Southeast Queensland, Australia, with her husband, their daughter, and the fat tabby cat, Ludo.